WOMEN *managing* STRESS

Other books by M. Sara Rosenthal

The Thyroid Sourcebook (4th edition, 2000)

The Gynecological Sourcebook (3rd edition, 1999)

The Pregnancy Sourcebook (3rd edition, 1999)

The Fertility Sourcebook (3rd edition, 1999)

The Breastfeeding Sourcebook (3rd edition, 1999)

The Breast Sourcebook (2nd edition, 1999)

The Gastrointestinal Sourcebook (1997; 1998)

The Type 2 Diabetic Woman (U.S. only; 1999)

The Thyroid Sourcebook for Women (1999)

Women and Depression (2000)

Women of the '60s Turning 50 (Canada only; 2000)

Women and Passion (2000)

Managing PMS Naturally (2001)

The Canadian Type 2 Diabetes Sourcebook (Canada only; 2001)

The Hypothyroid Sourcebook (2002)

50 Ways Series

50 Ways to Prevent Colon Cancer (2000)

50 Ways Women Can Prevent Heart Disease (2000)

50 Ways to Manage Ulcer, Heartburn and Reflux (2001)

50 Ways to Manage Type 2 Diabetes (U.S. only; 2001)

50 Ways to Prevent and Manage Stress (2001)

50 Ways to Fight Depression without Drugs (2002)

SarahealthGuides

These are M. Sara Rosenthal's own line of health books dedicated to rare, controversial or stigmatizing health topics you won't find in regular bookstores. SarahealthGuides are available only at online bookstores such as amazon.com. Visit **sarahealth.com** for upcoming titles.

Stopping Cancer at the Source (2001)

Women and Unwanted Hair (2001)

WOMEN *managing* STRESS

a sourcebook of natural solutions

m. sara rosenthal

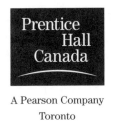

Prentice
Hall
Canada

A Pearson Company
Toronto

National Library of Canada Cataloguing in Publication Data

Rosenthal, M. Sara
   Women managing stress : a sourcebook of natural solutions

Includes index.
ISBN 0-13-043267-9

1. Stress management for women. I. Title.

RA785.R672 2002   155.9'042'082   C2001-903674-4

ISBN 0-13-043267-9

Editorial Director, Trade Division: Andrea Crozier
Acquisitions Editor: Nicole de Montbrun
Production Editor: Catherine Dorton
Copy Editor: Judith Turnbull
Proofreader: Liba Berry
Art Direction: Mary Opper
Cover Design: Mary Opper
Interior Design: Amy Harnden / Mary Opper
Cover Image: Larry Dale Gordon / The Image Bank
Author Photograph: Greg Edwards
Production Manager: Kathrine Pummell
Page Layout: Dave McKay

This publication contains the opinions and ideas of its author and is designed to provide useful advice in regard to the subject matter covered. The herbs and other treatments in this book are described for the information and education of readers. They are not a replacement for diagnosis and treatment by qualified health professionals. While every effort has been make to ensure its accuracy, the book's contents should not be construed as medical advice. Each person's health needs are unique. The author and publisher are not engaged in rendering health or other professional services in this publication. This publication is not intended to provide a basis for action in particular circumstances without consideration by a competent professional. The author and publisher expressly disclaim any responsibility for any liability, loss, or risk, personal or otherwise, which is incurred as a consequence, directly or indirectly, of the use and application of any of the contents of this book. To obtain recommendations appropriate to your particular situation, please consult a qualified health provider. The herbal information in this book is provided for education purposes only and is not meant to be used without consulting a qualified health practitioner who is trained in herbal medicine.

ATTENTION: CORPORATIONS
Books are available at quantity discounts with bulk purchase for educational, business, or sales promotional use. For information, please email or write to: Pearson PTR Canada, Special Sales, PTR Division, 26 Prince Andrew Place, Don Mills, Ontario, M3C 2T8. Email ss.corp@pearsoned.com. Please supply: title of book, ISBN, quantity, how the book will be used, date needed.

Visit the Pearson PTR Canada Web site! Send us your comments, browse our catalogues, and more.
www.pearsonptr.ca

1 2 3 4 5 WEB 06 05 04 03 02

Printed and bound in Canada.

A Pearson Company

Contents

Acknowledgments

I wish to thank the following people, listed alphabetically, whose expertise and dedication helped to lay so much of the groundwork for this book: Gillian Arsenault, M.D., C.C.F.P., I.B.L.C., F.R.C.P.; Louise Dorfman, counsellor and therapist, Couple Enrichment Inc.; Debra Lander, M.D., F.R.C.P.C., assistant professor of psychiatry, University of Manitoba; Mark Lander, M.D., F.R.C.P.C, associate professor of psychiatry, University of Manitoba, and a member of the Mood Disorders Clinic, Health Sciences Centre, Winnipeg, Manitoba; Sheila Lander, L.P.N./R.N., psychiatric nurse practitioner, Health Sciences Centre, Winnipeg, Manitoba; James McSherry, M.B., Ch.B., F.C.F.P., F.R.C.G.P., F.A.A.F.P., F.A.B.M.P.; Suzanne Pratt, M.D., F.A.C.O.G.; Donna Stewart, M.D., F.R.C.P., Lillian Love Chair in Women's Health, University Health Network and University of Toronto; Judith Ross, Ph.D., clinical psychologist and special lecturer, Department of Psychology, University of Toronto; David Rubinstein, M.A., counsellor and therapist, Couple Enrichment Inc.; Wm Warren Rudd, M.D., F.R.C.S., F.A.C.S., colon and rectal surgeon and founder and director of the Rudd Clinic for Diseases of the Colon and Rectum (Toronto); and Robert Volpe, M.D., F.R.C.P., F.A.C.P.

William Harvey, Ph.D., LL.B., University of Toronto Joint Centre for Bioethics, whose devotion to bioethics has inspired me, who continues to support my work and makes it possible for me to have the courage to question and challenge issues in health care and medical ethics. Irving Rootman, Ph.D., former director, University of Toronto Centre for Health Promotion, continues to encourage my interest in primary prevention and health promotion issues. Helen Lenskyj, Ph.D., professor, Department of Sociology and Equity Studies, Ontario Institute for Studies in Education/University of Toronto, and Laura M. Purdy, Ph.D., have been central figures in my understanding of the complexities of women's health issues and feminist bioethics.

Meredith Schwartz, my editorial assistant, and Larissa Kostoff, my editorial consultant, worked very hard to make this book come into being. And finally, Nicole de Montbrun, my editor at Prentice Hall Canada, championed this project and saw how important it was that all these health issues come together for this pervading women's health concern.

Introduction: What Is a Woman's Stress?

When you have written over 20 books in less than 10 years, you know a thing or two about stress. But it doesn't mean you know how to manage it.

I was 37 when I had my first panic attack—a freak occurrence, I thought, until the second one hit me. In this second case, I had been upset over a personal issue and had been crying non-stop for 48 hours. My aunt coaxed me out for brunch, and after our meal we decided to go to a fashion show at a nearby mall. While I watched the show, my mind wandered to my personal problem. Then I started to feel the same physical sensations I had experienced during my *first* panic attack a few months earlier: heart beginning to race, cold sweat, extreme dizziness, and nausea.

I said to my aunt, "Oh no—I think I'm having a panic attack; I have to get to a bathroom *now*." Try finding a bathroom in a busy Ontario mall! As we started on our odyssey, extreme dizziness and vertigo hit me. The next thing I remember was a voice: "Can you *hear* me? Can you *hear* me?" I opened my eyes and discovered I was lying on the floor of the mall, a crowd of people surrounding me. I couldn't see my aunt, but a kind woman, a stranger, was speaking to me: "It's okay; you just fainted. Just stay down for a minute." As I gathered my wits, I realized with great embarrassment that I'd been sick to my stomach.

After a few minutes I was helped up and escorted to the bathroom by a group of women; by this time, my aunt had reappeared (she had run to a phone to dial 911 and summon an ambulance). The ambulance crew brought a stretcher right into the bathroom, put me on it, and rushed me to the hospital. On the stretcher, I felt the vertigo return, and I began to throw up again. I also realized that my skills as a bioethicist were completely useless in my utter dependence on the ambulance atten-dant. I even said in a mocking tone: "And would you believe I'm a bioethicist?" "Informed consent" doesn't seem to matter very much when you're completely disoriented and the ceiling won't stop spinning.

Eventually, I did calm down, and I was released from the hospital that night. Later, I found out that had it not been for the kind public health nurse who just happened to be on the scene, I would have been in danger of aspirating vomit and dying. The message was clear: *my emotional stress was now becoming manifested as physical symp-*

toms. More to the point: *I had almost died from stress.* As a cancer survivor, I'm no stranger to facing my own mortality. But this was different. This was my wake-up call. Something had to change. I fainted on a Sunday and I called a therapist on the Monday.

Because I have written books on women and depression and know a fair bit about the subject, I was adamant about seeking out a therapist with a woman-centred approach who shared my views on antidepressants (I'm skeptical and critical about the mass dispensing of antidepressants to women) and who also shared my view that women have always had to squeeze themselves into a male-constructed world—a world that is not really built for women's minds and bodies. I was fortunate in my search. The first thing my therapist said to me was that panic attacks manifest themselves in two distinct ways, both of them physical metaphors for how we feel emotionally. People whose panic attacks take the form of vertigo—like mine did—feel their world is collapsing. Indeed, that weekend I felt exactly that way, and my body echoed those feelings. People whose panic attacks take the form of gasping for air and an inability to breathe—like several women I know—feel they have too much weight (as in responsibility) on their shoulders, and their bodies echo how they feel.

While I may be the author of this book, I am also its audience. I am not writing this from an ivory tower but from the rubble of a tower that collapsed. For me, managing stress is about gaining deeper insights into what stresses me out and finding ways to change my responses to stress and the lifestyle patterns that aggravate it.

This leads to a simple question with a complex answer: *what is a woman's stress?* In the story I just shared with you, I had an extreme physical reaction to emotional stress. (As I will explain in later chapters, *emotional stress* relates to something in your life that upsets you: relationships, finances, etc. *Physical stress* refers to stress that puts a strain on your body: occupational hazards, long commutes, sleep deprivation, etc.)

Many of the women I have spoken to about stress say that they live with an ongoing anxiety and "brimming" panic most of the time. Many, alternatively, develop full-blown episodes of depression, becoming disengaged from their lives. This is their bodies' way of tuning out stressors. Stress, depression, anxiety, and panic are interconnected. You can't separate them. An acknowledgment of this truth is perhaps what is new about my approach to stress in this book. Instead of attempting to separate stress as an isolated phenomenon, I argue that it is so much a part of being a woman that most women are not even aware of how much it affects them until their bodies tell them so. Allergies and asthma, back pain, high blood pressure, fatigue, digestive disorders, headaches, immune suppression (predisposing us to viruses, such as colds and flu, infections, autoimmune disorders, and cancer), and a host of other health problems can all be triggered by stress.

I began researching this book by collecting stories and narratives of women dealing with stress. Before long I recognized general patterns that have more to do with how women are socialized in Western culture, how our culture is structured and organized, and less to do with individual circumstances. Women are still working in professions that remain "pink ghettos": the majority of nurses, child-care workers, home-care and community-care workers, teachers, and administrative workers (receptionists, secretaries, etc.) are still women. More recently, "call centre" jobs can be categorized as pink ghettos, as 70 percent of these jobs are filled by women. Pink ghetto jobs are notorious for poor salaries, overwork, overtime, and, most stressful of all, a lack of *moral agency*—which means that the worker has no decision-making powers, often having to perform tasks that her instincts tell her are wrong.

Women in pink ghettos frequently rely on public transit to get to and from work. The risk of violence that goes with travelling alone on public transit late at night or walking unaccompanied in dangerous neighbourhoods, poorly lit areas, or areas that are notorious for acts of rape or assault (parking garages, parks) is another major source of stress for women that largely goes unnoticed and unreported.

When women have no moral agency in their jobs and are overworked and poorly paid, they can suffer from burnout. Burnout is the last phase of continuous stress resulting from job dissatisfaction and overwork. Signs of burnout include low morale, exhaustion, poor concentration, feelings of helplessness, depression, and disconnection from one's friends and family, the sense of being non-productive, and physical problems such as bowel problems, poor appetite, cramps, headaches, and so on.

Another chief cause of burnout is caregiving. Burnout tends to be highest in the caring professions, where workers are constantly exposed to non-stop suffering. In these cases, burnout has been described as a feeling of being spiritually drained, meaning that all one's energy is being poured into meeting the needs of others, leaving little left to fulfil one's own needs. The feeling of being used up emotionally and of having no control over one's work is an important distinction between burnout and depression. Some articles refer to burnout as "carers' fatigue" (defined as a hemorrhaging of oneself for others), suggesting that this is a long-known problem among both non-professional and professional women caregivers. In Canada, non-professional caregivers are responsible for 80 to 90 percent of the assistance provided to elderly persons in their homes, and the majority of caregiving is provided by women. No national policy addressing family members caring for elderly relatives exists at this time. Non-professional caregivers of the elderly are currently saving

Canada's health-care system more than $5 billion annually. Taxpayers would have to pay 276,509 full-time employees to do the work of the 2.1 million non-professional caregivers now providing the service.

Women continue to be under-represented in top corporate jobs and in the fields of science and technology, while government programs that may encourage young women to enter more challenging or academic careers are inadequate and hampered by existing social problems that make women the principal caregivers—for both adults and children—in our culture.

Stress affects women's bodies in unique ways, most of them not adequately covered in the reams of stress-management books available. That is because most research on stress is based on studies that have focused on the effects of stress on men. For example, one recent study reported by Time Health Media found that women are more likely than men to react to stress with a nurturing impulse, looking after others before themselves. This has been dubbed the "tend and befriend" response. Women need to understand the causes of stress from both the outside-in and the inside-out; they also need to see how stress affects them from the inside-out and outside-in. There are gender differences in both the causes and effects of stress, and there are unique social causes of stress for women that have to do with our positions in this culture. This book validates that fact, and allows the voices of women managing stress to be heard. The first step in managing stress is recognizing it. If you can see it, you can do something about it.

STRESS SYMPTOMS

You may be suffering from stress but don't know it. This section looks at how stress is manifested physically and emotionally.

1
THE PHYSICAL SIGNS OF
A WOMAN'S STRESS

Generally, stress is defined as a negative emotional experience associated with biological changes that allow you to adapt to it. In response to stress, your adrenal glands pump out *stress hormones* that speed up your body: your heart rate increases and your blood sugar levels rise so that glucose can be diverted to your muscles in case you have to "run." This is known as the "fight or flight" response. These hormones, technically called the catecholamines, are broken down into epinephrine (adrenaline) and norepinephrine.

The problem with stress hormones in the 21st century is that the fight or flight response isn't usually necessary, since most of our stress stems from interpersonal situations rather than from being chased by a predator. Occasionally, we may want to flee from a bank robber or mugger, but most of us just want to flee from our jobs or our kids! In other words, our stress hormones actually put a physical strain on our bodies and can lower our resistance to disease. Initially, stress hormones stimulate our immune systems, but after the stressful event has passed, they can suppress the immune system, leaving us open to a wide variety of illnesses and physical symptoms.

Hans Selye, considered the father of stress management, defined stress as the wear and tear on the body. Once we are in a state of stress, the body adapts to the stress by depleting its resources until it becomes exhausted. As we age, the wear and tear on our bodies mounts; we can suffer from the following stress-related conditions:

- Allergies and asthma
- Back pain

- Cardiovascular problems
- Dental and periodontal problems
- Depression
- Fatigue
- Gastrointestinal problems (digestive disorders, bowel problems, and so on)
- Headaches
- Herpes recurrences (especially in women)
- High blood pressure
- High cholesterol
- Immune suppression
- Insomnia
- Loss of appetite and weight loss
- Muscular aches and pains
- Premature aging
- Sexual problems
- Skin problems and rashes

Addictions and substance abuse, the potential result of attempts to self-medicate, may fuel many of these problems (see Chapter 3).

Current statistics from the Duke Center of Integrative Medicine reveal that 90 percent of women ignore clear physical signs of stress. While the list above indicates long-term effects of stress, the physical signs that you're under stress *now* include a fast pulse; shorter, gasping breaths; high, tight-sounding voice; tight upper back and neck; cold, clenched hands; and curled toes.

Since 43 percent of all adults suffer from health problems directly caused by stress and 75 to 90 percent of all visits to primary-care physicians are for stress-related complaints or disorders, the number of women who are not reporting physical problems related to stress is probably quite substantial.

Based on what *is* reported, about a million people per day call in sick because of stress, which translates into about 550 million absences per year in the traditional workplace. Other studies show that roughly 50 percent of all North American workers suffer from burnout—a state of mental exhaustion and fatigue caused by stress. Meanwhile, 40 percent of employee turnover is the direct result of stress.

The financial toll of occupational stress on North American industry adds up to about $300 billion annually; this figure was arrived at by factoring in absenteeism, lower productivity, employee turnover, and direct medical, legal, and insurance fees. California employers, for example, spend about $1 billion for medical and legal fees due to stress. Ninety percent of job stress lawsuits are successful, paying out four times that of other injury claims. Meanwhile, expenditures on stress management programs grew from $9.4 billion in 1995 to $11.31 billion in 1999. A more subtle but compelling statistic is this: in 1997 the Japanese word *karoshi*—"sudden death from overwork"—was found in English dictionaries.

Types of Stress

Managing your stress is no easy feat, particularly since stress comes in different forms. There are two basic types: acute stress and chronic stress.

Acute stress is the result of an acute situation, such as a sudden, unexpected negative event or an out-of-the-ordinary responsibility, such as having to organize a wedding or plan for a conference. When the event passes, the stress also passes. You experience acute stress when you're feeling the pressure of a particular deadline or event. There are numerous symptoms of acute stress: anger or irritability, anxiety and depression, tension headaches or migraines, back pain, jaw pain, muscular tension, digestive problems, cardiovascular problems, and dizziness.

But acute stress can also be *episodic*, meaning that there is one stressful event after another, creating a continuous flow of acute stress. A person who is always taking on too many projects at once is someone who suffers from episodic acute stress. Workaholics and those with the so-called Type A personality are classic sufferers of episodic acute stress.

I sometimes refer to acute stress as the "good stress" because good things often come from this kind of stress, even though it feels stressful or bad in the short term. This is the kind of stress that challenges us to stretch ourselves beyond our capabilities; it's what makes us meet deadlines, push the "outside of the envelope," and invent creative solutions to our problems. Examples of good stress include challenging projects; positive life-changing events (moving, changing jobs, or ending unhealthy relationships); confronting fears, illness, or people who make us feel bad (this is one of those bad-in-the-short-term/good-in-the-long-term situations). Essentially, whenever a stressful event triggers emotional, intellectual, or spiritual growth, it is a good stress. It is often not as much the event as it is your *response* to the event that determines whether it is a good or bad stress. The death of a loved one can sometimes lead to personal growth because we may see something about ourselves we did not see before—a new resilience, for example. A death, then, can be a good stress, even though we grieve and are sad in the short term. Regardless of whether acute stress is good or bad, it causes a surge of the hormone epinephrine, which increases the production of blood platelets, necessary for clotting. Unfortunately, an increase in platelets can also lead to blood clots, which can increase your risk of heart attack or stroke. Epinephrine also appears to thicken blood, raising the risk of heart attack and stroke even more.

What I call the "bad stress" is known as *chronic stress*. Chronic or bad stress results from boredom and stagnation, as well as prolonged negative circumstances. Essentially, when no growth occurs from the stressful event, it is bad stress. When negative events don't seem to yield anything positive in the long term, but more of the *same*, the stress can lead to chronic and debilitating health problems. This is not to say that we can't also get sick from good stress, but when nothing positive comes from the stress, it has a much more negative effect on our health. Some examples of bad stress include stagnant jobs or relationships, disability from terrible accidents or diseases, long-term unemployment, chronic poverty, racism, and lack of opportunities for change. These kinds of situations can lead to depression, low self-esteem, and a host of physical illnesses.

Within the larger categories of acute and chronic stress, stress can be defined in even more precise ways:

- Physical stress (physical exertion)
- Chemical stress (when we're exposed to a toxin in our environment; this would include substance abuse)
- Mental stress (when we take on too much responsibility and begin to worry about all that has to be done)
- Emotional stress (when we are stressed out by feelings such as anger, fear, frustration, sadness, betrayal, bereavement)
- Nutritional stress (when we are deficient in certain vitamins or nutrients, have overindulged in fat or protein, or experience food allergies)
- Traumatic stress (caused by trauma to the body, such as infection, injury, burns, surgery, or extreme temperatures)
- Psycho-spiritual stress (caused by unrest in our personal relationships or belief system, personal life goals, and so on. In general, this is what defines whether we are happy.)

Stress-Related Immune Suppression

Have you ever noticed how your body seems to ward off colds and flus while you're madly trying to meet some project deadline, and then the day you hand it in, you get hit with a terrible cold? Most studies show that stress hormones temporarily boost our immune system during a stressful event so that we're protected from illness while we have to perform. But after the stressful event has passed, the immune system defences plummet, leaving us immune suppressed. Over time, immune suppression can lead to very serious illnesses, not just garden variety colds and flus. Autoimmune diseases such as thyroid disease, lupus, multiple sclerosis, and so on—which develop in women at least 10 times more frequently than in men—are all related to immune suppression. Autoimmune disease means that your body creates antibodies to attack its own organs or functions, causing disease to develop. Cancers, for example, develop when people are immune suppressed. Pregnancy can also predispose women to autoimmune diseases. When you're pregnant, your immune system is suppressed to avoid destroying the developing fetus, which is foreign tissue. In the first three months of pregnancy and the first three months after delivery, women are at highest risk of developing an autoimmune disorder. Stress is a major factor in this statistic, as many women find they are completely unprepared for what's in store for them after giving birth.

> After I delivered my daughter, I started to feel extremely tired and sort of depressed. My doctor called it the "baby blues" and told me it would pass. Weeks of feeling tired and dragged out passed. I was also bloated and sort of "puffy" all over, and I finally asked my doctor to check me for other problems. I was diagnosed with Hashimoto's disease, which I was told was "autoimmune." My body apparently began attacking my thyroid gland, causing it to become inflamed and malfunction. I had to go on thyroid medication. I asked my doctor what caused it, and she asked me if I had been under any unusual stress lately. Having a baby was the most stressful event I can ever recall.

At least 20 percent of all new mothers will develop thyroid problems, while women under general stress can also develop thyroid disease. Because of limited space, this book cannot possibly cover the vast amount of material on autoimmune diseases. For more information on this subject, see *Living Well with Autoimmune Disease* by Mary J. Shoman.

Colds

We tend to shrug off colds as nothing serious, and we even continue to work and push ourselves when we're clearly sick. Women, especially, feel as though they can't give themselves permission to be sick and take care of themselves. But even the common cold, when not taken seriously, can lead to other health problems, as this story shows:

> I left my old job on a Friday and started my new job the following Monday with no time off in between. I was burning the midnight oil to finish a number of projects at the old job, and I was quite stressed. I woke up Sunday feeling really sick; I had a terrible cold. I figured it was my body trying to tell me to stop. Only I couldn't. I bought a bunch of cold medications at the drugstore and dragged myself into the new job on Monday. I just kept taking the cold medications and tried to deny that what I needed to do was go to bed. The cold just wouldn't get better, and I felt sicker and sicker as the week wore on. The following Monday, I went to see my doctor and discovered that I had developed "acute bacterial sinusitis"—a sinus infection—which I did not think was so cute. I asked my doctor if this was serious and she told me that unless I went on antibiotics, it could lead to "bacterial meningitis"! I took the antibiotics. Then I developed a yeast infection that wouldn't go away, as well as diarrhea, which I was told was caused by the antibiotic (an overgrowth of some gut bacteria was the cause). I've never felt so sick and dragged out in my life. I worked myself into such a poor state of health, something had to change. I asked for time off after only three months, and it was frowned upon. I wound up leaving the job just to take the time off I should have negotiated before changing jobs. I often ask myself whether I could have prevented several months of illness if I just taken 48 hours off and gone to bed. Guess I'll never know the answer. Now when I have a cold, I call in sick.

The Common Cold

You've all had it; you all know what it feels like; you all know the symptoms. What many of you don't realize is that the common cold can lead to a host of more serious health problems

Sinus Infections.

When a common cold has lasted for 7 to10 days and is no better or worse, acute bacterial sinusitis may have developed, which needs to be treated with antibiotics. If it remains untreated, you can develop chronic sinus disease, eye infections, bacterial meningitis, and even a brain abscess. Roughly 90 percent of all cases of bacterial sinusitis are cured with antibiotics. Decongestants are useless for sinus infections because they only open nasal passages, not the passages that drain the sinus itself, since these small passages are encased in bone.

Ear Infections.
Colds can also turn into acute bacterial middle-ear infections; this is more likely in children, but it can occur in adults, too. During colds, the tube from the back of the throat to the middle ear (Eustachian tube) can become swollen, obstructed, and infected. The result is a painful earache and temporary hearing loss. Like bacterial sinus infections, bacterial middle-ear infections can lead to mastoids and meningitis.

Worsening of Chronic Bronchitis.
Bronchitis is a bad cough accompanied by sputum, shortness of breath, and possibly a fever. The common cold can make this condition worse, but it won't usually cause bronchitis per se. But if you fall prey to a cold while combatting bronchitis, you can feel quite sick for many days.

Asthma Attacks.
If you suffer from asthma, a cold can trigger asthma attacks—particularly in children. All the more reason to read on!

Avoiding Colds

If you know that someone has a cold, avoid touching him or her, and wash your hands before you touch your nose or eyes. There are also a number of herbal treatments that can stop a cold before it starts, or fully "implodes," in your body.

Zinc.
Available as a lozenge. One zinc lozenge dissolved under the tongue at the first sign of a cold can stop it in its tracks according to years of anecdotal reports. (I, too, have great success using zinc.) A study published in the *Annals of Internal Medicine* that looked at zinc lozenges and the common cold in 48 patients showed that zinc lozenges reduced the severity and duration of the cold by almost 50 percent. Not all studies on zinc show the same results, but there are problems with the design of many studies looking at herbal products (see Chapter 10).

Echinacea.
Available in gel caps, tea, and extract. Echinacea is a popular prophylactic (meaning "preventive") cold remedy. Anecdotal evidence shows that taking echinacea at the first sign of a cold can either stop it before it becomes full-blown or shorten its duration. Studies looking at echinacea are difficult to design because three difference species of

echinacea are used as herbal medicines. Echinacea is also available in different preparations and strengths. (Recently, I caught what I thought would be a terrible cold. I drank three large cups of echinacea tea, went to bed at 8:00 p.m., and woke up feeling completely well!)

Zinc Nasal Spray.
Sold under the brand name Zicam. A study of 213 patients published in *ENT, the Ear, Nose and Throat Journal* found that Zicam nasal spray reduced cold symptoms by as much as 75 percent.

Aromatherapy.
(See Chapter 10.)

Critics of herbal cold cures make one good point: everyone recovers from the common cold anyway, so it's hard to know what the impact of the herbal cold cure truly is. If you had a mild cold that was going to get better on its own in three days and you took a zinc lozenge on Day 2, it's difficult to tell whether it was the lozenge or the natural lifespan of the cold virus that made you better by Day 3. That said, herbal cold cures won't hurt you, so you might as well try them unless your doctor specifically advises against them for some reason.

Over-the-Counter (OTC) Cold Medicines

Many of us survive colds with good old-fashioned OTC medications. Here's a list of these common remedies:

Antihistamines.
(See page 16.)

Non-steroidal Anti-inflammatory Drugs (NSAIDs).
Non-steroidal anti-inflammatory drugs (e.g., ibuprofen and naproxen) are good for reducing aches, pain, and fever. They block the production of certain natural inflammatory chemicals in our bodies called prostaglandins. NSAIDs are pretty useless for a stuffy nose and congestion, and there's no good reason to take them for these cold symptoms.

Decongestants.
If a bottle says "decongestant," it means that the product can open the nasal passages by shrinking blood vessels in the mucus membrane of the nose. (It's the swollen blood vessels that make you feel stuffed up when you have a cold.) Decongestants

come in all forms: liquid, pills, nose drops, and sprays. These drugs have side-effects and can speed up your heart, raise your blood pressure, or cause anxiety. If you're already under a lot of stress, you may want to rethink taking a decongestant.

Anticholinergics.

An anticholinergic is a drug that "dries you up." It helps reduce the amount of mucus in your nose. Unlike an antihistamine, this won't stop you from sneezing. Stay away from these if you have glaucoma. (Men with prostate problems shouldn't take them either.)

Cough Suppressants.

If you have a cough, you'll likely turn to these, but they can cause extreme drowsiness, so ask your pharmacist for a non-drowsy formulation. There are also cough syrups that loosen sputum so that you cough up "gunk," and there are other formulations for dry coughs. Don't make the mistake of buying the "sputum inducer" when you have a dry cough. Again, check with your pharmacist.

Sara's Chicken Soup for the Cold

I don't boast about too many things, but I am known for making really good chicken soup. When I'm under stress and have that "I'm-going-to get-sick-any-minute" feeling, I make my chicken soup and it helps me. This is the first time I've published this recipe, so I hope it helps you, too!

The first rule of chicken soup is this: if you're going to make it, make a *big* pot of it. That way you know it will be there for you if you do fall prey to a cold. Although I can't prove it, I believe my chicken soup has prevented illness many times. Chicken soup actually contains compounds that help to decrease congestion. When the soup is made with vegetables, the phytochemicals from the vegetables also contribute health benefits. A study conducted by a pulmonary specialist at the University of California, Los Angeles, found that a chemical called acetylcysteine (which is found in decongestants) functions similarly to the amino acid cysteine, which is abundant in the proteins in chicken soup.

Here's the recipe in seven steps (it has not been tested in a test kitchen):

1. Put raw chicken whole, or in parts, in a big soup pot/cauldron that can hold about 6 cups/1.5 L of water. (Any parts will do, but I favour thighs and legs.) A whole chicken needs at least 6 cups/1.5 L of water; 3–4 chicken parts need at least 4 cups. Alternatively, you can use the remains of chicken that was previously cooked.

2. Bring the pot to a boil. Don't cover. You will begin to see white stuff float to the top. (This is charmingly known as "soup scum.") Skim this off and discard. (Note: If the chicken was previously cooked, there will be no "white stuff.")

---

3. Add about 1 tablespoon/15 mL of salt and 1 chicken bouillon cube or packet. If the soup isn't salty enough for you once you taste it, add no more than another tablespoon of salt.

4. Add 1 large onion or 2 small onions, cut in quarters.

5. Add whole garlic cloves, at least 4 but stop at 8. (Garlic is known for its antibiotic, immune-boosting properties.)

6. When the white stuff has been removed and no more is floating to the top of the pot, add the following vegetables all at once: 4–5 carrots, chopped in large diagonal pieces (for some reason it tastes better that way and I don't know why!); 4–5 stalks of celery, also cut in diagonals (be sure to add the celery tops—the leafy things); 2–3 parsnips, also cut in diagonals; and fresh dill (very key!). If you don't like dill, use parsley.

7. Cover the pot. Reduce the heat to a simmer temperature and just leave the pot alone for at least an hour. I prefer to eat the soup "country bumpkin" style with pieces of chicken and vegetables in the bowl. For more elegance, you can strain out the veggies and chicken pieces, bones, etc., and eat as a broth; to liven up the plain broth you can put rice or pasta in it, such as tortellini. (Note: When you're feeling better, you can make risotto with the leftover broth.)

This soup can be refrigerated for up to a week and heated up in portions as needed. Freeze the rest after a week.

Flu

When you're immune suppressed, you're vulnerable to influenza, or the "flu." In a new era of bioterrorism, you may be inclined to shrug off the flu as not that serious compared to other infectious agents, but each year about 20,000 North Americans die because of flu-related pneumonia; about 90 percent of those deaths occur in the frail or elderly.

If you've been hit with the flu in the past, you know how miserable it can be. Generally, the flu vaccine (a.k.a. flu shot) is recommended for certain populations of people (see below). People who are immune suppressed are always advised to get a flu shot. If you've never had a flu shot and never seem to get the flu, you may not need to be vaccinated. But if you're undergoing a period of high stress, you may benefit from a flu vaccine.

The flu is essentially a respiratory tract infection that hits urban populations in the late fall, winter, or early spring. It is very contagious and spreads from person to person through the sprays emitted from coughing and sneezing. In 1918 one bad strain of the flu caused over 20 million deaths worldwide and 500,000 deaths in the United States. The 1968 Asian flu was responsible for over 50,000 deaths in the United States.

When you have the flu, you feel really sick. You may develop a sudden fever as high as 104°F, with shaking chills, muscle and joint aches, sweating, dry cough, nasal congestion, sore throat, and headache. Severe fatigue and just feeling horrible in general (called "malaise") always accompany these symptoms. The flu can keep you down for as long as two weeks; if you're lucky, you'll escape with a week. The main complication of the flu is pneumonia, which is what people wind up dying from when they're very frail or elderly.

If you want to avoid the flu, ask your doctor about getting a flu vaccine. People who should not be vaccinated are those with an allergy to chicken eggs; people who've had a previous bad reaction to the flu vaccine; or those who are currently ill with a fever. Generally, U.S. and Canadian flu advisory experts recommend that the following groups of people always get a flu vaccine:

- Anyone over 65 (the U.S. recommends anyone over age 50)
- Anyone living in a nursing home or long-term-care facility
- Anyone with chronic heart or lung disease
- Anyone with asthma or kidney disease
- Anyone with diabetes
- Anyone who is immune suppressed or immune compromised due to cancer treatment, HIV, organ transplants, steroid medications
- All health-care workers
- Anyone caring for someone vulnerable to the flu
- Children aged six months to eight years who are receiving long-term aspirin therapy (the flu in this case can lead to Reye's syndrome, a rare disorder)
- Pregnant women in the second or third trimester during flu season
- Anyone travelling abroad

There are now a number of homeopathic flu-prevention therapies you can ask your natural pharmacist about. Contact Canada's leading natural pharmacy, Smith's Pharmacy, for more information: **www.smithspharmacy.com**.

If you do come down with the flu, all you can do is ride it out with herbal/homeopathic treatments, aspirin, acetaminophen, or ibuprofen, which will help with aches, fever, and chills. Drink lots of liquids (the more you drink, the more you pee; the more you pee, the more you pee out the flu). Stay home and rest. If you live in Toronto, maybe I can send you some of my chicken soup.

Allergies and Asthma

Allergies and asthma are also worsened by immune suppression. Here's a tale about stress-related allergies that we can all relate to:

> Last year I was trying to get a mortgage as a self-employed single woman. Although I was pre-approved prior to making an offer on a house, once the bank received the offer, they said I didn't "qualify" for the mortgage because I was self-employed. (I say it was because I was a woman who was self-employed!) For over a month, I went through one banking institution after another looking for someone to finance me, almost losing the house I wanted to buy in the process. During that month, I suddenly developed terrible allergies to dust mites—something that never bothered me before. I couldn't stop sneezing and my nose was constantly stuffed. It became debilitating. When I finally got financing and the deal closed, my allergies mysteriously stopped. But now, every time I'm stressed, they flare up again.

It's not your imagination that more people—particularly women—are suffering from allergies. In addition to stress, exposure to workplace chemicals and toxins is also putting women at risk for occupational asthma and allergies, which can lead to chronic fatigue. According to the *Journal of the American Medical Association* (*JAMA*), at least 10 million North Americans suffer from chronic asthma and as much as 15 percent of asthma is the direct result of occupational exposure. One of the most notorious chemicals is toluene diisocyanate (TDI), a substance used in the plastics and oil industries. It is also found in factories where boats, recreational vehicles, and electronic products are manufactured.

Because of poor air circulation, high-rise office buildings are another source of asthma and allergies; this is known as "sick building syndrome." Ventilation systems can distribute throughout a building the mold that grows inside ducts, car exhaust when air intakes are placed in parking garages, bacteria from bird feces if birds nest in or around the vents, and asbestos fibres and fibreglass.

Also at risk for asthma and allergies are women who work with animals (the proteins in animal skin and urine can trigger asthma), health-care workers who have reactions to natural proteins in rubber latex gloves, and women who work in food plants and inhale dust from cereal protein and flour.

Many women notice a significant drop in their energy levels and endurance because of chronic asthma and allergies resulting from exposure to various man-made materials. A 10-year study by the National Institute for Occupational Safety and Health in the United States revealed that asthma is among the leading job-related diseases in the United States. Canada has similar statistics.

The following materials, common in homes and workplaces, have been cited as hazardous to your health and/or well-being. While they may not all be carcinogenic, many of the items on this list cause headaches, rashes, and asthmatic symptoms.

- Asbestos building materials
- Cleaning products and disinfectants
- Urea formaldehyde foam insulation
- Adhesives (may contain naphthalene, phenol, ethanol, vinyl chloride, formalde-hyde, acrylonitrile, and epoxy, which are all toxic substances that release vapours)
- Artificial lighting (can cause headaches)
- Toners used in copy machines and printers
- Particleboard furniture and space dividers
- Permanent ink pens and markers (contain acetone, cresol, ethanol, phenol, toluene, and xylene, which are toxic)
- Polystyrene cups
- Second-hand smoke
- Synthetic office carpet (may contain acrylic, polyester, and nylon plastic fibres, formaldehyde-based finishes, and pesticides due to moth-proofing for wool only)
- White-out correction fluid (may contain cresol, ethanol, trichloroethlyene, and naphthalene, which are all toxic chemicals)

Multiple Chemical Sensitivity (MCS)

This term was introduced in the early 1990s to explain a wide array of health prob-lems and symptoms that appear to be reactions to chemicals. Among the many differ-ent symptoms associated with MCS are depression and chronic fatigue, sleep disturbances, mood swings, and poor concentration. People considered at risk for MCS include those who

- work or live in energy-sealed buildings;
- are exposed to fumes from carpets, pesticides, cleaners, and airborne allergens;
- are exposed to industrial chemicals, such as those found in plants that process wood, metal, plastics, paints, and textiles;
- are in constant contact with pesticides, fungicides, and fertilizers;

- live in high-pollution areas; or
- work in dry cleaning, hair salons, pest control, printing, and photocopying.

Reproductive Concerns

Women, of course, want to protect their reproductive organs. We know, for example, that if you are a dental hygienist and work in an unventilated area, you may be overexposed to nitrous oxide, which is linked to high rates of miscarriage. If you are exposed to certain solvents, ranging from those found in dry-cleaning businesses to those used in the semiconductor industry, you may also be at risk.

Employers must make known to all employees in the workplace the existence of any chemical classified as "hazardous" by the appropriate government bodies, detailing the relevant components, hazards, and handling instructions specific to that chemical. This enables working mothers in particular to decide whether they want to stop working while pregnant or find work in a hazard-free environment. And, of course, these hazardous chemicals may interfere with breastfeeding. All foreign compounds that appear in your blood also appear in your breast milk. However, toxin exposure is less critical during breastfeeding than it is during pregnancy, especially during the early stages.

How Toxic Is This Stuff?

In Canada, the Toxicological Index database (Infotox) provides peer-reviewed information concerning workplace chemicals that may affect women's reproductive organs, especially during pregnancy and breastfeeding. There are also various drug and poison hotlines (listed locally) that have considerable information on toxins affecting pregnancy and breast milk. For more information, you can go to the National Institute of Occupational Safety and Health (NIOSH) website: **www.cdc.gov/niosh**. NIOSH Information Dissemination can also be accessed directly by calling (513) 533-8287. You can also consult the Centers of Disease Control and Prevention (CDC) in Atlanta at (404) 639-3311. Finally, you can contact the Occupational Safety and Health Administration (OSHA) by visiting **www.osha.gov**. OSHA is the federal agency in charge of worker safety and health.

Herbal Allergy Treatments

There are a number of homeopathic and naturopathic allergy treatments available, but they vary greatly on so many factors, including your allergy symptoms, that it's impossible to discuss them adequately here. Your lifestyle, diet, and overall exposure to various allergens should be assessed by a naturopathic or homeopathic practitioner before a remedy is suggested.

There are essential oils that help with allergies, the most popular of which is peppermint oil. If you're sneezing and congested, peppermint oil can be diffused in a room or applied directly to (this sounds weird) the nape of your neck, as well as to the skin over your thymus gland (at the indent in your neck at the front) and the soles of your feet. Do not apply peppermint oil to your nose or face, as it is very strong and can greatly irritate the skin. You can also add a few drops of peppermint oil to a hot bath. If you are allergic to dust mites, you can use peppermint oil as a dusting oil and apply it to wood—this is especially effective around your bed.

OTC Allergy Medications

Again, many people survive allergies by taking over-the-counter antihistamines. An antihistamine inhibits what's called a histamine, which is a natural inflammatory substance your body makes. Histamine is what causes you to sneeze, drip, and even cough. This isn't always a bad thing, but it's important not to use antihistamines for prolonged periods of time.

If you tend to suffer from allergies in sealed environments with poor air circulation, taking an antihistamine prior to airplane travel can save you from the pain of clogged sinus passages during takeoff and landing.

The first generation of antihistamines have a sedating effect and are better for colds than for allergies. The second generation of antihistamines—non-sedating—are what most people take today for allergies.

The sedating antihistamines are dangerous if you are trying to maintain other activities. Alcohol, sedatives, and tranquilizers will increase the sedating effect. Again, stay away from these if you have glaucoma (men with prostate problems should avoid them, too!).

Give Your Immune System a Boost

Stress lowers our resistance to disease by suppressing our immune systems. Here's an overview of some of the more well-known immune boosters, substances that stimulate or strengthen your immune system to help it fight diseases, including cancer:

Echinacea.
Echinacea is a flower that belongs to the sunflower family. Also mentioned under herbal cold cures, this immune booster is not just for colds. It's believed that echi-

nacea increases the number of cells in your immune system to help you fight off diseases of all sorts.

Essiac.
Essiac is a mixture of four herbs: Indian rhubarb, sheepshead sorrel, slippery elm, and burdock root. Essiac is believed to strengthen the immune system, improve appetite, supply essential nutrients to the body, possibly relieve pain, and, ultimately, prolong life.

Ginseng.
Ginseng is a root used in Chinese medicine; it's believed to enhance your immune system and boost the activity of white blood cells.

Green Tea.
Green tea is a popular Asian tea made from a plant called *Camellia sinensis*. The active chemical in green tea is epigallocatechin gallate (EGCG). It is believed that green tea neutralizes free radicals, which are carcinogenic. It is considered to have anti-cancer properties—particularly for stomach, lung, and skin cancers.

Iscador (a.k.a. mistletoe).
Iscador is made through a fermentation process that uses different kinds of mistletoe, a plant known for its white berries. More popular as an anti-tumour treatment in Europe, Iscador is believed to work by enhancing your immune system and inhibiting tumour growth.

Pau d'Arco (a.k.a. Taheebo).
Pau d'arco usually comes in the form of a tea made from the inner bark of a tree called Tabebuia. Pau d'arco is believed to be a cleansing agent and can be used as an antimicrobial agent; it is said to stop tumour growth.

Wheatgrass.
Grown from wheatberry seeds, wheatgrass is rich in chlorophyll. Its juice contains over 100 vitamins, minerals, and nutrients, and is believed to contain a number of cancer-fighting agents and to have immune-boosting properties.

The following spices are said to be "tumour busters":

- Garlic
- Turmeric
- Onions

- Black pepper
- Asfetida
- Pippali
- Cumin and poppy seeds
- Kandathiipile
- Neem flowers
- Mananthakkali, drumstick, and basil leaves
- Ponnakanni
- Parsley

Headaches

Headaches are one of the chief complaints women have when they are under stress. They are caused by a variety of factors, so it's not surprising that there are different kinds of headaches with different symptoms. If you suffer from headaches, the first order of business is to determine whether they are migraine or non-migraine headaches. If you suffer from migraine headaches, see further on in this section for information. If your headaches are non-migraine headaches, read on!

Tension Headache

This is the classic stress-induced headache, and it is manifested as a pressure or aching in the head. Fatigue and hunger (both of which can be aggravated by stress) can also cause this type of headache. Women in their 30s are the most likely sufferers of tension headaches. However, women are also more likely to experience tension headaches at certain times in their reproductive lives. Pregnant women and women with new babies tend to suffer from tension headaches, as do women going through menopause. Which aspect of this is hormonal and which is due to the stresses of going through significant life changes is hard to determine.

Overall, since the causes of tension headaches are stress, fatigue, and hunger, they can be relieved by relaxation, rest, and food. If you can't find the time for food, rest, or relaxation, you can try a natural remedy, such as an essential oil (see Table 10.1), or take acetaminophen, aspirin, or ibuprofen. If you are pregnant or breastfeeding, do *not* take anything for your headache—herbal or otherwise—without first consulting your health-care provider or the MotherRisk hotline: (416) 813-6780.

Tension headaches are more common in women than in men, affecting about 42 percent of the female population. They can last several hours or even days, and tend to affect both temples at the front of the head. The pain is usually not severe but takes the form of a dull aching, which can range in severity from mild to moderate. Tension headaches are either episodic (they do not bother you more than 15 days per month) or chronic (they occur more often than 15 days per month). Women with chronic tension headaches may also be battling with depression (see Chapter 2).

Some headache experts believe that tension headaches are a less severe form of migraine headaches, but this is only a working theory. Since tension headaches can also be brought on by high blood pressure, they may indeed be a precursor to migraines, which are caused by restricted blood flow.

Cluster Headache

A cluster headache begins suddenly with a pain that is short, sharp, and severe; it is much more common in men than in women; and it often goes away fairly quickly. It is more of a "headache attack" than a gradual onset of pain, and it is called a cluster headache because the attacks come in clusters over several days or weeks. You may also have several attacks per day. Cluster headaches are caused by an expansion of the blood vessels, which is why the pain is severe and throbbing. These headaches strike without warning and can last for only 15 minutes or as long as three hours. Pain on one side of the head, around the eye or temple, eye redness, eye watering, constricted pupil, or a drooping eyelid on the "headache side" are other symptoms of cluster headaches. The pain is so severe that it is difficult to sit still during an attack; sweating and congestion can also occur in response to the pain.

Two of the main causes of cluster headaches are smoking and alcohol. When you're stressed, you may smoke and/or drink more to self-medicate, so in a roundabout way, stress may significantly contribute to cluster headaches. Weather changes and changes in sleep patterns can also bring on attacks.

The main treatment approach for cluster headaches is prevention. Cutting down on cluster headache triggers such as smoking and alcohol is the least invasive approach. Finding a way to stop the attack when it first strikes is the next treatment option. In this case, there are some strong medications that your doctor can prescribe or you can experiment with various over-the-counter medications, such as ibuprofen, acetaminophen, or aspirin.

Sinus Headache

Sinus headache is caused by inflammation of the sinuses, or *sinusitis*. It is not caused by stress per se, but since stress can affect your immune system and leave you more vulnerable to infection, if you're prone to sinus infections, you may get more of them when you're stressed. A symptom of a sinus headache is pain around the cheekbones and forehead and behind the eyes. Since sinuses drain into the nose, when they're inflamed, the pressure and pain follow the nasal passages, resulting in pain in the upper face, behind the eyes and nose. Cigarette smoke (either yours or second-hand), weather changes, or other allergy triggers can bring on a sinus headache—especially if you suffer from allergies. Allergies can also be triggered by stress, which is another link between stress and sinusitis.

Treating a sinus headache involves treating the sinus infection. Thick yellowish-green mucus in the nose is a surefire indicator of a sinus infection. Antihistamines or decongestants may help relieve the headache, since they help relieve congestion. Many doctors over-prescribe antibiotics for sinus infections; this would be a route in an extreme case, but antibiotics can lead to antibiotic resistant sinus infections, which are nastier.

Rebound Headache

If you've been taking pain relievers for headaches over the course of several days, you may find that your headache returns when the pain medication wears off. In this case, you need to wean yourself off the medication because your body is now dependent on it and your headaches may be withdrawal headaches.

> I started taking Tylenol for what I thought was a normal stress headache. The headache would disappear for a while but would then reappear. I found that unless I took Tylenol every four hours or so, the headache would just loom. This went on for a couple of weeks. I once got addicted to nasal sprays and figured out that it was the spray that was causing my chronic nasal congestion. I thought the same thing might be going on with the headaches. I went to a health food store and asked if they could recommend something "natural" for a headache, and I was told that marjoram, an essential oil, was good for headaches. It took a few days before the headache disappeared, but now I avoid all headache medications and try to ride it out with natural therapies and massage.

The medications most responsible for rebound headaches are the ones that contain caffeine, but any headache medication taken more than three days per week can cause rebound headaches. Taking medications at higher doses than is recommended on the package or by your doctor can also lead to rebound headaches. For example, taking four pills every two hours when the label advises "two pills every six hours" can lead to dependence and rebound headaches. Many people start at the recommended dose and increase their dosage as the headache persists or worsens. Often a higher dose is necessary to produce the same results that the lower dose once did. But if you need to take higher doses to relieve the same quality and level of headache, you've probably become dependent on the drug. Headaches that persist while you're on medication or that return when the medication wears off are indications of medication dependence and rebound headaches. Side-effects of the medication may also lead to a headache, producing a "which came first" scenario.

Treating rebound headaches involves abstaining from the headache medication and using alternatives to treat the headache, such as massage, essential oils, and so on.

Secondary Headache

This type of headache develops as a side-effect of another health problem. If you are over 50 and are noticing a new kind of headache, one you've never had before, go to your health-care provider to rule out other conditions that may be causing the headache. Treatments will vary depending upon the underlying cause of this type of headache. Common causes of secondary headaches include the following:

- Anemia (meaning that you are low in iron)
- Glaucoma (the headache would be caused by increased pressure within the eye)
- Temporomandibular joint disorder (TMJ—a misalignment of the jaw)
- Increased pressure in the brain (for a number of reasons)
- Tumour (many of these are benign)
- Subdural hematoma (when blood accumulates between the two outer membranes of the brain)
- Infection
- Stroke
- Inflamed arteries
- Head injury
- Overexertion

Secondary headaches tend to be severe, and they almost always feel "new" in the sense that you won't recall having felt this way before. If nausea, vomiting, fever, or drowsiness accompanies this headache, it is especially alarming and you should get yourself to an Emergency Room right away.

Migraine Headaches

Migraines are the nuclear weapons in the headache arsenal. Most people believe that migraine headaches are stress-related, but the research is divided about this. The only thing we know for sure about the subject of migraine headaches, women, and stress is that women report that they suffer from more migraines while under stress. What does the science say? We know that migraines are caused by dilated blood vessels and that dilated blood vessels are triggered by low levels of serotonin. Migraines are also influenced by the menstrual cycle, and we now know that lower levels of estrogen can affect serotonin levels. When estrogen levels fall, so do serotonin levels. Women tend to suffer from migraines before their periods (migraines are commonly linked to PMS), during their first trimester of pregnancy (although they are usually migraine-free during the second and third trimesters, when estrogen levels are very high), and around menopause. Women plagued by migraines probably started having them around the time of their first period (a.k.a. menarche). The relationship between stress and migraine headaches, then, quite probably has to do the ways various stressors affect serotonin levels and the menstrual cycle. Migraines usually don't just "erupt" or develop in people who don't have a history of migraine headaches. But if you have a history, stress can definitely trigger more episodes. Many more women than men suffer from migraines (18 percent of women compared to 6 percent of men).

The subject of migraines is so huge that migraines have been broken down into subcategories. Migraines are considered a separate category of headache because for those suffering from them, it is almost like living with a debilitating disease. While in the throes of a migraine attack, most people cannot function at all and are confined to bed, in a dark room.

A migraine headache is more than a throbbing pain on one side of the head (the pain can be moderate or severe); other symptoms tag along:

- Nausea and/or vomiting
- Aversion to light (a.k.a. photophobia)
- Aversion to sound (a.k.a. phonophobia)

- Aversion to movement (this is why most people lie very still—the movement worsens the pain)
- Aversion to certain smells or tastes
- Aversion to touch

In short, the symptoms that accompany the migraine headache are actually due to a heightening of all the senses (taste, touch, smell, sight, and sound).

Some people experience "auras" before a migraine attack. These can take the form of flashing or pulsating squiggles of light or just floating spots. The aura may last anywhere from 5 to 60 minutes, and it disappears before the headache begins. For many, this is a warning to take preventive measures (adjusting their schedules) or take preventive medication. Numbness and difficulty speaking can also accompany the migraine. This is what's known as the *classic migraine*, and it affects about 15 percent of the migraine population. People who do not experience auras have *common migraine*, which affects about 85 percent of migraine sufferers.

The pain in the head is caused by an expansion of blood vessels rather than a constricting of blood vessels (what normally happens with headaches). Many headache medications, or any medication that dilates blood vessels, can make the migraine worse.

Migraine headaches are also linked to more serious problems, such as epileptic seizures, strokes (27 percent of all strokes suffered by people under 45 are related to migraines), aneurysms, permanent vision loss, severe dental problems, and even coma. The point of telling you this is not to scare you, but to emphasize that migraines are extremely serious. Women sufferers often feel that their employers or co-workers shrug off their migraine complaints as trivial. Many people do not understand that migraines can be incapacitating, requiring time off.

Migraine Triggers

Unavoidable migraine triggers are fluctuating hormone and serotonin levels, which can be influenced by many factors, including strong emotions and stress. Changes in atmospheric pressure and high altitudes can also trigger migraines. Weather is such an enormous trigger that Canada conducted a study on it, concluding that the following weather patterns can increase the likelihood of a migraine attack:

- A drop or change in barometric pressure
- The passing of a warm front
- Heat and humidity or a high humidex

- Rain
- Southeast winds

But there are also avoidable triggers, such as red wine, scotch, aged cheeses, caffeine, nicotine, oversleeping, or fatigue. Other avoidable triggers include bright light, strong chemical smells (imagine if you worked in a lab!), second-hand smoke, fish (this can dilate blood vessels), some chocolate, and foods that contain nitrates or MSG.

By combining your knowledge of weather patterns and avoidable triggers, you can control migraine attacks to some extent. For example, you can take preventive medications during certain weather conditions. (Many medications don't work, so please discuss this with your doctor; there are also medications that work only at certain times.) Most people practise evasive manoeuvres (avoiding stress as much as they can, adjusting their schedule, etc.) when they know they're vulnerable to a migraine.

Headache Diaries

If you're plagued by either migraine or non-migraine headaches, experts suggest that you keep a headache diary. The following information should be recorded in this diary:

1. Where are you in your menstrual cycle?

2. What did you eat in the last four hours?

3. What is the weather pattern?

4. What level of stress were you experiencing prior to the headache?

5. What medications did you take before, during, and after your headache?

6. How much sleep did you get last night?

7. What other symptoms accompanied your headache (e.g., nausea, dizziness, etc.)?

By recording these seven pieces of information, you will see a pattern to your headaches and be able to determine how much stress is involved in triggering them. You may also be able to identify those things that commonly trigger your headaches. Once identified, these triggers can be avoided during times of high stress.

Stress-Related "Bathroom Blues"

The signs of stress aren't always visible in your mood or disposition. Your body may be reacting to stress much more than you realize. Irritable bowel syndrome (IBS) and interstitial cystitis (IC) are disorders that mostly affect women, and they are believed to be triggered by stress. Thus, by reducing your stress, you may be able to find significant relief from these disorders.

Hazards of Not Being Able to Go to the Bathroom

My boss asked me to step into his office one day, and he told me that he noticed too many "absences" from my desk. Embarrassed, I told him that I do need to go to the ladies' room frequently, especially when I'm under stress. I didn't want to elaborate. Afterwards, I started to feel really self-conscious and would avoid going to the bathroom, even when I really had to go. I felt watched all the time and didn't feel comfortable just going when I felt like it. I guess I held in my urine too much, because I started getting bladder infections. Finally, I confronted my boss and told him that I did not feel it was appropriate to be made to ask permission to go to the ladies' room when I was over 40! The situation did not improve, and he constantly referred to my "absences" as in: "I was looking for you a while ago and couldn't seem to find you anywhere …" I quit that job because of my bathroom habits, and that makes me very angry.

Sometimes bathroom-related stress is caused by the stress of not being able to get to a bathroom. Hats off to the ABCNews program *20/20* for exposing one of the most ignored occupational hazards women put up with daily: not enough, or poorly designed, bathrooms on the premises. Well, here's a news flash for business and industry: women have a uterus that presses down on the bladder, biologically necessitating more frequent urination. Frequency increases, of course, with pregnancy, fibroids, and other below-the-belt nuisances women endure. Heavy periods often necessitate frequent trips to the bathroom, too. Being forced to "hold it in" is unhealthy physically *and* psychologically. Physically, women are at high risk for developing urinary incontinence, urinary tract infections, and interstitial cystitis, which is associated with chronic pelvic pain, frequent urge without "results," and sometimes incontinence.

The most shocking indication of the pervasiveness of this bathroom problem comes from *20/20*'s report on the practices of a Fortune 500 company. In one of its central plants in the U.S., the company had provided only a *single* toilet for its more than 100 female employees. The women didn't have enough time on their breaks to wait in line and go to the bathroom. The penalty for coming back from the break "late" was lost pay. The result was that many of these women were forced to wear incontinence briefs (a.k.a. adult diapers) just so they could continue working without being tormented by the urge to urinate.

Restraining the urge to defecate has some nasty health hazards for women, too. For example, many more women than men are diagnosed with irritable bowel syndrome, a condition caused by stress and often characterized by diarrhea. Many women also suffer from inflammatory bowel disease, which also leads to frequent bouts of bloody, mucus-filled diarrhea; this problem, too, may be aggravated by stress and menstrual flow.

The psychological damage of these practices on women is, of course, enormous. When grown women are forced to wear diapers, they suffer from low self-esteem, unexpressed anger, and a myriad of negative feelings and thoughts that can trigger the symptoms of depression discussed in Chapter 2.

In many workplaces, as the tale that opened this section suggested, women have to ask permission of their superiors to go to the bathroom. Again, this infantilizes women and should not be tolerated. More women than men work in "visible yet vulnerable" occupations (as receptionists or in secretarial/assistant positions); getting up and leaving their desk is sometimes just not doable. In these cases, adequate "coverage" from a second or third person should be provided. Many women report that their superiors note the number of times they go to the bathroom. These "logs" are used to the women's detriment in performance reviews, in the form of criticism for "frequent absences from the desk." If you can relate to this section, it's worth noting how much aggravation and stress are added to your day simply because you don't feel at liberty to go the bathroom when you need to. I'll touch on workplace issues more in Chapter 5.

Irritable Bowel Syndrome

A most confusing label has come into vogue, one that defines the bowel habits of between 25 and 55 million North Americans, two-thirds of whom are women. The label—*irritable bowel syndrome* (IBS)—refers to unusual bowel patterns that alternate between diarrhea and constipation, and include everything in between. IBS is also referred to as irritable or spastic colon; spastic, mucus, nervous, laxative, cathartic, or functional colitis; spastic bowel; nervous indigestion; functional dyspepsia; pylorospasm; and functional bowel disease. The problem with using the term "irritable" is that irritation is *not* what's going on. It also sounds too much like "inflammatory," which is not what's going on either. Worse, many family doctors will say, "You've got IBS," instead of "We don't know what's going on—but have you tried fibre?"

The term *irritable bowel syndrome* came into use to describe a bowel that is overly sensitive to normal activity. When the nerve endings that line the bowel are too sensitive, the nerves controlling the gastrointestinal tract can become overactive, making the bowel overly responsive or "irritable" to normal things, such as passing gas or fluid. In other words, the bowel may want to pass a stool before it's time. The bowel, in a sense, becomes too "touchy" for comfort. However, since we tend to associate the word "irritable," when used clinically, with something that is red, irritated, or inflamed, this label is more confusing than defining. IBS has nothing to do with irritation, inflammation, or any organic disease process. It has to do with nerves.

The term IBS also implies that a diagnosis of your symptoms has been made and that there is a definite cause—and cure—for your condition. This is not so at all. IBS is a diagnosis made in the absence of any other diagnosis. There is no test to confirm IBS, only tests to rule out other causes of your symptoms. The term *functional bowel disorder* is beginning to catch on instead of IBS, because "functional" means that there is no disease. Yet no matter what you call it, roughly half of all digestive disorders are attributed to IBS. After the common cold, IBS is the chief cause of absenteeism. Many doctors compare IBS to asthma in that there are a number of causes with the same outcome. Asthma may be related to allergies or to a hundred other things. Similarly, IBS has many different causes that are difficult to pin down. However, stress and dietary factors are the chief causes.

IBS Symptoms

IBS symptoms are characterized by frequent, violent episodes of diarrhea that will almost always strike around a stressful situation. (People often experience IBS symptoms before job interviews or plane trips.) Over 60 percent of IBS sufferers report that their symptoms first coincided with stressful life events; 40 to 60 percent of people with IBS also suffer from anxiety disorders or depression, compared to 20 percent of people with other gastrointestinal disorders. Stressful life events that can bring on IBS include death of a loved one, separation/divorce, unresolved conflict or grief, moving to a new city or job, as well as having a history of physical or sexual abuse in childhood.

Many people will find that their symptoms will persist well beyond the stressful life event and that the episodes will invade their normal routine. There need not be one single stressful event that precipitates IBS; the condition could first present itself after you have worked in a stressful job for some time or have been subjected to the normal stresses of life in North America for a long period. The episodes of diarrhea are often accompanied by crampy, abdominal pains and gas, which are relieved by a bowel movement. The pain may shift around in the abdomen as well. After the diarrhea episodes, you may then be plagued by long bouts of constipation or the feeling that you're not emptying your bowels completely when you do go. Again, IBS refers to an irregular bowel *pattern* rather than one particular episode. The pattern is that there is no *normal* pattern of bowel movements; it is often one extreme or the other.

Your stool may also contain mucus, which can make the stool long and rope-like or worm-like. The mucus is normally secreted by the colon to help the stool along in a normal movement. In IBS, your colon secretes too much mucus. Blood mixed with your stool means that this is not IBS, but something else. Some people can also suffer from diarrhea alone or solely from gas and constipation. Other symptoms include bloating, nausea, and loss of appetite. Fever, weight loss, and severe pain are *not* signs of IBS; they indicate some other problem.

Many people find it confusing that IBS can cause both constipation and diarrhea, since these seem to be at opposite ends of the spectrum. But what happens is that instead of the slow muscular contractions that normally move the bowels, spasms occur, which can result in either an "explosion" or a "blockage." It's akin to a sudden gust of wind; it can blow the door wide open (diarrhea) or blow it shut (constipation). It all depends on the direction of the wind at the time. It's important to note the timing of your diarrhea; in IBS, your sleep should not be disturbed by it. The episodes will always occur either after a meal or in the early evening.

You can tell that you are suffering from IBS rather than infectious diarrhea or inflammatory bowel diseases if you

- find relief through defecation;
- notice looser stool when the bowel movement is precipitated by pain;
- notice more frequent bowel movements when you experience pain;
- notice abdominal bloating or distention;
- notice mucus in the stool; or
- feel that you have not completely emptied your bowels.

What to Rule Out

The symptoms of IBS are obviously a little inconclusive in that they can be signs of many other problems. Therefore, before you accept a diagnosis of IBS, make sure your doctor has taken a careful history to investigate the following other possible diagnoses:

- Dietary culprits, food allergies, lactose intolerance, or just plain poor diet—high fats/starch, low fibre
- Intestinal bacterial, viral or parasitic infections (where have you been travelling? what are your sexual habits?)
- Overgrowth of *C. difficile*, a common cause of infectious diarrhea
- Yeast in the gastrointestinal tract (called candidiasis), which is notorious for causing IBS symptoms (eating yogurt every day should clear this up)
- Medications
- Gastrointestinal disorders, such as dysmotility, where the stomach muscles are not moving properly, causing bloating, nausea, and other problems
- Enzyme deficiencies (the pancreas may not be secreting enough enzymes to break down your food)
- Serious disease such as inflammatory bowel disease or cancer

Stress and IBS

It's possible to have a pristine diet, rule out all forms of organic disease, and still suffer from IBS while under stress. In the same way that you can sweat, blush, or cry under emotional stress, your gastrointestinal tract may also react to stress by "weeping"—producing excessive water and mucus, overreacting to normal stimuli such as eating. What often happens, however, is that there is a delayed gut reaction to stress, and you may not experience your IBS symptoms until your stress has passed. Apparently, under stress your brain becomes more active so that you can better defend yourself. (For example, when you're running away from a predator, you have to think and act quickly, so your heart rate increases, you sweat more, and so on.) During this defensive mode, the entire nervous system can operate in an exaggerated way (that's what causes "butterflies in the stomach"). The nerves controlling the gastrointestinal tract therefore become highly sensitive, sometimes causing IBS symptoms. Studies show, for example, that IBS symptoms are more common on weekday mornings than afternoons or weekends and that they don't appear at night while you're sleeping.

Women and IBS

Why is IBS more common in women? For one thing, women menstruate and thus experience normal mood fluctuations related to their natural menstrual cycles. Mood changes are common premenstrual symptoms that may create emotional stress, and hence, IBS symptoms. Another factor is uterine contractions during menstruation. When the uterus contracts, it often stimulates a bowel movement. Women often have several loose bowel movements on the first day of their period. (A common symptom of labour is diarrhea and vomiting. This occurs because of the intensity of the uterine contractions, which create "ripples" throughout the gastrointestinal tract.)

Women who experience painful periods or endometriosis may also experience IBS symptoms more intensely. In endometriosis, parts of the uterine lining grow outside of the uterus, into the abdominal cavity, often triggering painful bowel movements, diarrhea, or constipation during or just prior to menstruation.

Finally, women are much more prone to eating disorders and laxative abuse, as well as being the more likely victims of domestic abuse (resulting in continuous emotional upset and stress), all of which wreak havoc on the gastrointestinal tract.

Bladder Problems

Another stress-related condition women suffer from is *interstitial cystitis* (IC), which is the inflammation of the interstitium, the space between the bladder lining and bladder muscle. This can cause chronic pelvic pain, urinary frequency, and a shrunken, ulcerated bladder. The bladder itself is lined with a protective layer that is secreted, like mucus, by the cells that line the bladder. This layer protects the inside of the bladder from acids and toxins in the urine and prevents bacteria from sticking to the bladder wall. If this layer is damaged, as is the case with IC, infection can result.

IC symptoms include frequent urination (as many as 60 times per day). In addition, you may feel a bruising kind of pain around your clitoral area and may find that acidic foods, chocolate, red wine, old cheese, nuts, yogurt, avocados and bananas—and sometimes, antibiotics—seem to make the pain the worse. IC starts out as a normal urinary tract infection (known as bacterial cystitis), but after a few bouts of cystitis, the urine cultures will all be negative.

There are several theories about the causes of IC, including one that identifies increased progesterone levels as the culprit. In fact, postmenopausal women on progesterone may notice cystitis symptoms more than premenopausal women. If you have IC, you'll need to see a urologist. There are numerous treatments, including anti-inflammatory drugs and bladder relaxants.

Improving Bladder Control or Incontinence

Note: Roughly 75 percent of women will experience one or more incidents of urinary incontinence after menopause. This may result in *stress incontinence* (leakage when laughing, sneezing, coughing, picking something up, running, and performing any other normal activity that puts stress on the bladder). It may also be experienced as *urge incontinence* (leakage as soon as the urge comes on, except there is no time to get to the toilet). Damaged or weakened pelvic-floor muscles (often a consequence of childbirth) are the cause. Other aggravating factors include alcohol use, urinary tract infections, fibroids, and chronic constipation.

Avoid the following bladder irritants:

- Caffeine
- Alcohol
- White sugar
- Citrus
- Tomatoes
- Cayenne
- Hot peppers
- Iced drinks
- Carbonated drinks
- Pineapple
- Cigarettes (smoking increases your risk of developing stress incontinence by 350 percent)
- Certain common medications: diuretics, antidepressants, beta-blockers, blood pressure–lowering drugs, sleeping pills, tranquilizers

Herbal Remedies

- Pulsatilla
- Zincum
- Boil dried teasel (*Dipsacus sylvestris*) roots with 1 tablespoon/15 mL to 1 cup/250 mL of water for 10 to 15 minutes, and then drink daily.
- Replace your coffee with cranberry juice.
- Antispasmodic herbs such as black cohosh, ginger, catnip, and cornsilk may control incontinence.

- Yarrow (*Achillea milefolium*) will help heal bladder infections, incontinence, and heavy periods, but may aggravate hot flashes. Recommended as a tea or infusion of the dried flowers as desired, or as a tincture of the fresh flowering tops, 5–10 drops, 2–3 times daily.

Conventional Remedies

- Hormone Replacement Therapy (HRT) and estrogen vaginal creams are highly effective in reversing incontinence caused by vaginal and bladder wall thinning.

Bladder Control Exercises

- To tone vagina and bladder: Sit in a bathtub with water up to your hips. See if you can suck water into your vagina and expel it. Suck in as you breathe in; push out as you breathe out. Do this 25 to 50 times.
- Kegel exercises: Isolate the tiny muscles that start and stop your urinary stream. (In other words, next time you pee, stop the flow.) Hold as long as you can (work up to at least 10 seconds) before letting go and peeing again. Practise this every time you urinate. (You can also do this when you're not urinating, to strengthen the muscle.)
- Pulse your urine flow by pushing out very strongly, then slackening it off until it's just a dribble, then pushing out again, and so on. Repeat as many times as possible every time you urinate.
- Empty the bladder completely every time you void by pressing down behind your pubic bone with fingertips or the flat of your palm.
- Scheduled toileting: Pee on a regular schedule, say, every 60 to 90 minutes. After three to four consecutive dry days, increase the interval by 15 to 30 minutes and keep increasing until you're at every four hours.

Stress-Related Insulin Resistance

Stress can affect how well your cells respond to the hormone *insulin*. Insulin is a major player in your body, and one of its most important functions is to regulate your blood sugar levels. It does this by knocking on your cells' door and announcing: "Sugar's here; come and get it!" Your cells then open the door to let sugar in from your bloodstream. That sugar is absolutely vital to your health, providing you with the energy you need to function. When the cell doesn't answer the door, this is called *insulin resistance:* the cell is resisting insulin. What happens if the cells don't answer the door? Two things. First, the sugar in your bloodstream will accumulate because it has nowhere to go. (It's the kind of situation that develops when your newspapers pile up outside your door when you're away.) Second, your pancreas will keep sending out more insulin to try to get your cells to open that door. This results in high blood sugar. The end result is too much sugar and too much insulin, a bad combination of problems that can lead to high blood pressure (a.k.a. hypertension), high cholesterol, and a host of other complications.

The way blood sugar works is pretty complicated. It gets even more complicated if you're a woman. That's because estrogen influences your blood sugar levels and insulin requirements. There is also evidence that estrogen-containing products can trigger insulin resistance in women who have a family history, or genetic predisposition, to Type 2 diabetes. (Type 2 diabetes used to be called adult onset diabetes, a completely different disease than Type 1 diabetes, which used to be called juvenile diabetes.) Estrogen usually *raises* blood sugar levels. This is why estrogen-containing medications, such as oral contraceptives or hormone replacement therapy, were once considered no-no's for women with diabetes. It is also why diabetes is still labelled a *contraindication* (meaning a condition that is not compatible with a given therapy or medication) for many estrogen-containing products.

If you've noticed the following symptoms, you should have your blood sugar tested and be screened for Type 2 diabetes:

- Weight gain. When you're not using your insulin properly, you may suffer from excess insulin, which can increase your appetite. This is a classic Type 2 symptom.
- Blurred vision or any change in sight. There is often the feeling that your prescription eyewear is weak.
- Drowsiness or *extreme* fatigue at times when you shouldn't be drowsy or tired
- Frequent infections that are slow to heal. Women should be on alert for recurring vaginal yeast infections or vaginitis, which means vaginal inflammation, characterized by itching and/or foul-smelling discharge.
- Tingling or numbness in the hands and feet
- Gum disease. High blood sugar affects the blood vessels in your mouth, causing inflamed gums; the sugar content can get into your saliva, causing cavities in your teeth.

Diabetes experts also point to the following as possible signs of Type 2 diabetes in women.

- Irregular periods, such as changes in cycle length or flow
- Depression, which could be a symptom of either low or high blood sugar
- Headaches (from hypoglycemia)
- Insomnia and/or nightmares (from hypoglycemia)
- Spots on the shin (known as necrobiosis diabeticorum)
- Decaying toenails
- Muscle pains or aches after exercise (high blood sugar can cause lactic acid to build up, which can cause pain that prevents you from continuing exercise)

Stress-Related Fatigue

> Ever since I had my children, I can't remember not feeling exhausted all the time. I run on about five hours of sleep. I sometimes feel that I'll never know my former energy levels again. By the time I get the kids ready for school and off for their day, I barely have time to get myself out the door to work. I race to the daycare to get the kids (they charge extra for each five minutes you're late after 6:00 p.m.), get dinner ready, get them to bed. I don't want to go to bed at that point; I want to have time to do something for me, even if it's watching reruns on television. I find that I linger until about 1:00 a.m., and then I'm further behind in sleep. It's been this way for at least three years.

Fatigue is one of the most common complaints doctors hear from their patients. Most women have multiple roles, juggling career and family pressures. If you're over 40, chances are you have an ailing parent that you have to care for on top of your own family. I discuss this more in Chapter 4. The point to be made here is that there is a difference between feeling normal stress-related fatigue and feeling chronic fatigue, which is characterized by low energy, lethargy, and flu-like symptoms. This section outlines some of the factors responsible for normal fatigue. Generally, normal fatigue can be remedied by making some lifestyle changes.

Sleep Deprivation

Women with demanding jobs that require long hours are often sleep deprived. This is a problem that can have serious health repercussions. Recent research has found that not only does sleep deprivation deplete the immune system (it depletes you of certain cells needed to destroy viruses and cancerous cells), but it can promote the growth of fat instead of muscle and may speed up the aging process.

This happens because lack of sleep increases levels of the hormone cortisol, which is the stress hormone. As cortisol levels rise, the muscle-building human-growth hormone and prolactin (a breastfeeding hormone that also helps to protect the immune system) both decrease. Normally, during sleep, cortisol levels decline, while the human-growth hormone and prolactin increase. Cortisol also declines prior to sleep, as this is the body's way of preparing for sleep. Cortisol normally increases in the morning to make you more alert. It is also released by the adrenal gland in response to stress; essentially, it is an "alert" hormone that makes you take action. It explains why you are alert during important meetings, are up to "closing the sale or deal," or suddenly become incredibly articulate with someone on the phone after spending five days with two toddlers without any relief. The hormone will subside in the body as the stressful event passes.

A common reason women in particular cut down on their sleep is that they want to get in their "workout time" before their day begins. It's not unusual for many working women to rise at 5:00 a.m. in order to get their exercise. This, according to sleep experts, only *compromises* health and increases stress. The benefits of the exercise may be cancelled out by the harm done by lack of sleep. In the United States, a National Sleep Foundation survey revealed that two out of three people get less than the recommended eight hours of sleep per night; of that group, one out of three gets less than six hours of sleep.

There are two phases of sleep: rapid eye movement (REM) and non-rapid eye movement. It's during REM sleep, researchers believe, that we dream, an important component in mental health. Non-REM sleep is when we are in our deepest sleep, and it's then that various hormones are reset and energy stores are replenished.

It's estimated that, right now, roughly 50 percent of people diagnosed with depression get too much REM sleep and not enough deep, replenishing, non-REM sleep.

Sick Kids

In the film *As Good as It Gets,* Helen Hunt portrayed a Manhattan waitress who had to look after her asthmatic child in an urban environment. Hunt won at Oscar for her role, and working mothers with similar responsibilities openly cheered in theatres as she expressed her frustration with the lack of social supports for mothers and sick children. Few women can escape the stresses involved with the "second shift," another term used for the "double duty" problem, especially when there's a shortage of affordable child care in North America. When children get sick or suffer from chronic health problems such as asthma or allergies, women often must run their child back and forth to doctors, miss work, and miss sleep. Due to a decline in our air quality, the incidence of childhood asthma and allergies has skyrocketed; this places working mothers in a difficult position, as they are usually the parent that cares for the sick child. Childhood asthma is often misdiagnosed as something else, which can lead to high doses of expensive and unnecessary medication and added financial stress.

We are also seeing more chronic ear infections in children and more childhood cancers. Again, all this places tremendous stress on mothers and contributes to extreme sleep deprivation and fatigue.

Abnormal Fatigue: Chronic Fatigue Syndrome

Seventy percent of all people who suffer from chronic fatigue are women under the age of 45. *Chronic fatigue syndrome* (CFS) has been around longer than you might think. In 1843, for example, a curious condition called "fibrositis" was described by doctors as being characterized by symptoms now seen in *fibromyalgia* (chronic muscle and joint aches and pains) and chronic fatigue syndrome (symptoms of fibromyalgia accompanied by flu-like symptoms and extreme fatigue). The term *rheumatism*, an outdated label, was frequently used as well to describe various aches and pains with no specific, or identifiable, origin.

In the late 1970s and early 1980s, a mysterious virus, known as the Epstein-Barr virus, was being diagnosed in thousands of young, upwardly mobile professionals, at the time known as "Yuppies"—the baby boom generation. People were calling this condition the Yuppie flu, the Yuppie virus, Yuppie syndrome, and burnout syndrome. Many medical professionals were stumped by it, and many regarded it as a phantom or psychosomatic illness. Because so many women were dismissed by their doctors as hypochondriacs or were not believed to be ill or fatigued, the physical symptoms triggered self-doubt, feelings of low self-esteem, self-loathing, and so on; these feelings in turn often triggered depression. But even with the most sensitive medical attention, depression seems to go hand in hand with CFS simply because the disorder leaves so many sufferers at home in bed, isolated from the active lifestyle so many of them once had. In other words, some believe that in the case of CFS, depression is a normal response to "feeling like hell" every day of your life! This is an example of the "if you weren't depressed, you'd be crazy" adage I began to use as I researched this book.

A lot of people with CFS have been misdiagnosed with various diseases that shared some of the symptoms we now associate with CFS. These diseases include mononucleosis, multiple sclerosis, and HIV-related illnesses (once called AIDS-related complex, or ARC), Lyme disease, post-polio syndrome, and lupus. If you were diagnosed with *any* of the above diseases, please take a look at the established symptom criteria for CFS below. You, too, may have been misdiagnosed.

In the early 1980s, two physicians in Nevada treated a number of patients who shared a curious condition (after a nasty winter flu had hit the region). The doctors identified this condition as "chronic fatigue syndrome"— perhaps its most accurate label and the one that has stuck. But there are other names for CFS, such as the U.K. label M.E. (which stands for myalgic encephalomyelitis) and postviral fatigue syndrome. CFS is also known as chronic fatigue immune deficiency syndrome (CFIDS), because it's now believed that CFS sufferers are immune suppressed, although this is still in debate. For the purposes of this chapter, I'll use the simpler label that seems to tell it like it is: chronic fatigue syndrome.

The Symptoms of CFS

The term *chronic fatigue syndrome* refers to a collection of ill-health symptoms (not just one or two), the most identifiable of which are fatigue and flu-like aches and pains.

It wasn't until 1994 that an official definition of chronic fatigue syndrome was actually published in the *Annals of Internal Medicine*. The Centers of Disease Control (CDC) have since published official symptoms of CFS, too. Although many physicians feel that the following list of symptoms is limited and requires some expansion for accuracy, it includes, as of this writing, the official defining symptoms of CFS:

- An unexplained fatigue that is "new." In other words, you've previously felt fine and have only noticed in the last six months or so that you're always fatigued, no matter *how* much rest you get. The fatigue is debilitating; you're not as productive at work and it interferes with normal activities—social, personal, and academic. You've also noticed poor memory or weak concentration, and this affects your activities and performance, too. *In addition to this fatigue, four or more of the following symptoms will have persisted for at least six months:*

  - Sore throat
  - Mild or low-grade fever
  - Tenderness in the neck and underarm area (lymph nodes in these areas may be swollen, causing tenderness)
  - Muscle pain (called myalgia)

- Pain along the nerve of a joint, without redness or swelling
- A strange and new kind of headache
- You sleep but wake up unrefreshed (a sign of insufficient amounts of non-REM sleep)
- You feel tired, weak, and generally unwell for a good 24 hours after you've had even moderate exercise

A Word about Exercise Tolerance

Some CFS experts feel that *poor exercise tolerance* (meaning that even modest exercise is followed by such exhaustion and malaise that you can't tolerate it) is perhaps the *hallmark* symptom of CFS. Some scientists researching CFS have suggested that there is indeed a biological reason for this that has to do with a deficient flow of oxygen and energy to your cells during exercise. Normally, oxygen increases in our bodies with exercise; in CFS sufferers, oxygen seems to decrease with exercise, which may explain a lot! Without oxygen during exercise, various "poisons" (accumulated substances we produce naturally, such as lactic acid, magnesium, etc.) can build up and reduce the efficiency of our tissues and organs. Why this seems to be happening remains to be discovered; *whether* it is happening at all still needs to be confirmed and further documented, according to many other scientists.

What Your Doctor Should Rule Out

Since there are so many causes of fatigue and malaise, before diagnosing CFS, your doctor should rule out the following:

- Multiple sclerosis
- An underactive thyroid gland (known as hypothyroidism)
- Sleep disorders (such as sleep apnea or narcolepsy)
- Side-effects from any medications you're taking
- Hepatitis
- Major depression or bipolar affective disorder that predates your symptoms (see Chapter 2)
- Eating disorders
- Substance abuse or alcohol abuse within two years of your current symptoms

- Obesity-related fatigue and malaise. If you're very heavy, a number of the symptoms of CFS could be related to your size. In this case, losing weight may help to resolve the symptoms.
- Lyme disease
- Sexually transmitted diseases, including HIV and syphilis
- Fatigue related to your menstrual cycle (fatigue is often a symptom of PMS and of estrogen loss as women approach menopause). Anemia, due to heavy menstrual flow, is an extremely common cause of fatigue.
- Pregnancy- or postpartum-related fatigue (see Chapter 4)
- Allergies. Delayed symptoms of an allergic reaction can be joint aches, pains, eczema, and fatigue. Foods and environmental toxins can be classic triggers.

If none of the above is responsible for your condition, you may be suffering from CFS. You may also be diagnosed with the frustrating label *idiopathic fatigue*, which means that your fatigue is of "unknown origin." This is not very helpful, and you should find out why you don't meet CFS criteria if your symptoms persist.

Fibromyalgia versus CFS

Fibromyalgia is a soft tissue disorder that causes you to hurt all over—all the time. It appears to be a condition that is triggered and/or aggravated by stress. If you notice fatigue and more general aches and pains, this suggests CFS. If you notice *primarily* joint and muscle pains, *accompanied* by fatigue, this suggests fibromyalgia.

Fibromyalgia is sometimes considered to be an offshoot of arthritis, and it's not unusual for it to be misdiagnosed as rheumatoid arthritis. Headaches, morning stiffness, and an intolerance to cold, damp weather are common complaints with fibromyalgia. People with this disorder also commonly suffer from irritable bowel syndrome or bladder problems.

Causes of CFS

There is no official known cause of CFS, but there are several theories related to everything from viral agents that infect the population to airborne environmental toxins and poisons that can damage the immune system.

Some CFS sufferers have an impaired immune system, similar to what happens with people infected by HIV. This suggests that there *may* be some viral agent(s) at work. But other CFS sufferers have an overactive immune system, indicating that CFS may be an autoimmune condition, meaning that the immune system is manufacturing antibodies that are attacking the body's own tissues. Autoimmune diseases are triggered by stress. The pain and inflammation many CFS sufferers report are more likely due to an overactive immune system, while the flu-like malaise and fatigue are more likely due to an underactive immune system. This is why CFS continues to remain a mystery to researchers. When a body is poisoned by environmental toxins, however, it's possible that different toxins can trigger different reactions in different immune systems, which may explain the paradox. Gulf War syndrome, for example, is characterized by a wide array of symptoms. Different bodies may also react differently to the same toxin.

Stress appears to be a major trigger of CFS. When we are under stress, our bodies produce the hormone *adrenaline*, which increases our heart rate, blood flow, blood pressure, and so on. Adrenaline may aggravate the inflammation and pain many CFS and fibromyalgia sufferers experience.

Some experts who treat CFS and fibromyalgia believe that a lack of non-REM sleep may also be a factor in these disorders. Some experts have gone on record to say that chronic fatigue syndrome is really a sleep-related disorder. In one Canadian study, a group of medical students were deprived of non-REM sleep over a period of several nights. Within the next few days, each of the study participants developed symptoms of CFS and/or fibromyalgia.

Treatments

Since experts agree that CFS is an environmental illness triggered by stress, an improved diet and lifestyle modification appear to be effective ways to treat CFS. Certain "trigger foods"—foods that typically trigger allergies or fungal (*Candida albicans*) infections (processed foods, foods high in sugar or yeast, etc.)—are eliminated and replaced with more nutritious vitamin-packed organic foods. Since so many CFS sufferers have Candida, adjusting the diet is a logical first step. Candida is a yeast-like fungus that normally inhabits our digestive tract. This parasite can overgrow and spread to other places in the body, damaging the immune system.

Often a move to a cleaner environment is useful (changing jobs or telecommuting if you believe you're being exposed to workplace toxins; moving from an urban centre to a suburb or rural area). "Downshifting," a term coined to describe people who simplify their lifestyles by getting away from the urban "noise and toys," has worked wonders in shedding stress. And you can often improve CFS by reducing your stress levels. This may involve moving to a smaller place, with a lower monthly payment, leaving a job, buying that farm you've always wanted, or just cashing in your RRSPs and taking a long trip. (This was known in the 1960s as "dropping out.")

CFS experts and fellow sufferers will caution you about taking antidepressants—often the first thing a medical doctor will prescribe. Since antidepressants have many side-effects that can aggravate CFS symptoms, they are reportedly not the best solution as a first-line treatment for CFS. The general advice is to try cleaning up your diet and lifestyle first and then see if your symptoms improve. Symptoms of depression in CFS often clear up when you start to feel a little better physically and get out of the house!

A number of alternative therapies are reported to work with CFS. Check out Part 3 of this book for starters. I hesitate, as of this writing, to recommend the treatments I came across in my research because they are simply not substantiated yet. But as with so many herbs and alternative therapies, ranging from glucosamine sulphate (for arthritis) to St. John's wort (for depression), the fact that they're not proven in traditional scientific studies doesn't mean they don't work. Time will tell, as well as word of mouth. To date, however, diet modification is the most effective treatment that CFS experts recommend, along with cognitive therapy, which is a type of counselling that helps you to shift your thinking or focus.

Stress-Related Cardiovascular Problems

The panic and anxiety that many women suffer while under stress can cause heart palpitations, but more insidious is stress-related hypertension, or *high blood pressure.* The blood flows from the heart into the arteries (blood vessels), exerting pressure against the artery walls. The simplest way to explain this is to think about a liquid-soap dispenser. When you want soap, you need to pump it out by pressing down on the little dispenser pump, the "heart" of the dispenser. The liquid soap is the "blood" and the little tube, through which the soap flows, is the "artery." The pressure that's exerted on the wall of the tube is therefore the "blood pressure."

When the tube is hollow and clean, you needn't pump very hard to get the soap; it comes out easily. But when the tubing in your dispenser gets narrower as a result of old, hardened, gunky liquid soap blocking the tube, you have to pump much harder to get any soap, while the force that the soap exerts against the tube is increased. Obviously, this is a simplistic explanation for the very complex problem of high blood pressure, but essentially, the narrowing of the arteries forces your heart to work harder to pump your blood. If this goes on too long, your heart muscle enlarges and becomes weaker, which can lead to a heart attack. Higher pressure can also weaken the walls of your blood vessels, which can cause a stroke.

The term *hypertension* refers to the tension or force exerted on your artery walls. (*Hyper* means "too much"—thus "too much tension.") Blood pressure is measured in two readings: X over Y. The X is the *systolic* pressure, which is the pressure that occurs during the heart's contraction. The Y is the *diastolic* pressure, which is the pressure that occurs when the heart rests between contractions. In "liquid soap" terms, the systolic pressure occurs when you press the pump down; the diastolic pressure occurs when you release your hand from the pump and allow it to rise back to its "resting" position.

In the general population, target blood pressure readings are 130 (or less) over 85 (or less)—that is, <130/85. Readings of 140/90 or higher are generally considered borderline, although for some people this is still considered a normal reading. For the general population, 140/90 is "lecture time," the time when your doctor will begin to counsel you about dietary and lifestyle habits. By 160/100, many people are prescribed a hypertensive drug, which is designed to lower blood pressure.

Let's examine some of the causes of hypertension. Hypertension is exacerbated by tobacco and alcohol consumption and too much sodium or salt in the diet. If high blood pressure runs in your family, you're considered at greater risk of developing hypertension. High blood pressure can also be caused by kidney disorders or pregnancy (known as pregnancy-induced hypertension). Medications are also common culprits. Estrogen-containing medications (such as oral contraceptives) and non-steroidal anti-inflammatory drugs (NSAIDs)—such as ibuprofen, nasal decongestants, cold remedies, appetite suppressants, and certain antidepressants—can increase blood pressure. Be sure to check with your pharmacist.

How to Lower Your Blood Pressure without Drugs

When your stress levels are lowered, your blood pressure will drop. So by reading this book, you're off to a good start! Here are some other ways to lower blood pressure:

- Change your diet and begin exercising.
- Limit your alcohol consumption to no more than 2 oz/57 g of liquor or 8 oz/227 g of wine or 24 oz/680 g of beer per day; for liver health, limit the amounts to even less.

- Limit your salt intake to about 1 1/2 teaspoons/7 mL per day by cutting out all foods high in sodium, such as canned soups, pickles, soy sauce, and so on. Some canned soups contain 1000 mg of sodium, for example. That's a lot!
- Increase your intake of calcium or dairy products and potassium (i.e., bananas). Some still-unproven studies suggest that people with hypertension are calcium- and potassium-deficient.
- Lower your stress levels. Studies show that by lowering your stress, you lower your blood pressure.

Herbs to Lower Blood Pressure

The following herbs can help to lower blood pressure:

- **Hawthorn.** As a tincture, 10–20 drops three times daily.
- **Motherwort.** As a tincture, 10–20 drops three times daily.
- **Dandelion root.** As a tincture, 10–15 drops with meals
- **Potassium.** Eighty to 85 percent of people who eat six portions of potassium-rich foods daily will reduce their need for blood pressure–lowering medication by half or more.
- **Raw garlic.** Just 1/2 to 1 clove of raw garlic a day can dramatically reduce your blood pressure. Mince it raw into a variety of dishes, including eggs, rice, and potatoes.
- **Ginseng.** Available in tea form or gel caps.
- **Seaweed**

Blood Pressure–Lowering Drugs

If you can't lower your blood pressure through lifestyle changes, you may be a candidate for some of the following blood pressure–lowering drugs:

Diuretics.

Diuretics are the most commonly used blood pressure medication. Also known as water pills, diuretics work by flushing excess water and salt (often 2–4 lbs/1–2 kg worth!) out of your system. But diuretics may actually increase the risk of heart attack by leaching potassium salts needed by the heart, and the heart may respond to blocked nerve signals by trying harder and harder until it fails. Another common side-effect of diuretic therapy is low potassium. Levels of potassium tend to drop when diuretics replace the low-fat diet you've worked so hard to maintain. If you make sure not to substitute one therapy for another, diuretics will not affect your potassium levels. Other side-effects include increased blood sugar and cholesterol levels.

Beta-blockers.

Beta-blockers alter the way hormones like adrenaline control blood pressure. They slow the heart rate by decreasing the strength of the heart's contractions. Beta-blockers are most often used by young people and/or people with coronary artery disease. Possible side-effects include fatigue and an increase in blood sugar and cholesterol levels.

Centrally Acting Agents.

These drugs act through centres in the brain to slow the heart rate and relax the blood vessels. Possible side-effects include stuffy nose, dry mouth, and drowsiness.

Vasodilators.

Vasodilators dilate, or relax, the blood vessels, thereby reducing blood pressure.

Ace-inhibitors.

Ace-inhibitors lower blood pressure by preventing the formation of a hormone called *angiotensin II*, which causes the blood vessels to narrow. Ace-inhibitors are also used to treat heart failure. Possible side-effects include cough and swelling of the face and tongue.

Alpha-blocking Agents.

Alpha-blocking agents block the effects of noradrenaline, a stress hormone, allowing the blood vessels to relax. Blood pressure decreases with treatment, as does cholesterol. You may also notice an increase in HDL, or "good" cholesterol. A possible side-effect is blood pressure variation when standing versus reclining.

Calcium-Channel Blockers.

Calcium-channel blockers limit the amount of calcium entering the cells, allowing the muscles in the blood vessels to relax. Possible side-effects include ankle swelling, flushing, constipation, and indigestion.

Heart Attacks in Women

I had this terrible heartburn last year, with other stomach pains. It was something I'd never felt before and I thought it was serious. I started to feel ill while I was at work, and I called my daughter to pick me up and take me to the Emergency Room.

I was seen by a very young resident or student (who knows anymore?) and was told that I was " fine" and sent home with a recommendation to take some Zantac. The next day, I called my own doctor, who sent me to a cardiologist. The cardiologist told me that I had had a mild heart attack, and asked me why I'd waited so long to come in. When I told the cardiologist what had happened at the ER, he shook his head and just said numbly, "This happens all the time, and I'm damned sick of it!"

Stress significantly contributes to heart disease in women. First, stress causes women to smoke, which can lead to heart disease. It also contributes to high blood pressure and insulin resistance, which in turn can lead to diabetes, high cholesterol, and obesity—all major risk factors in heart disease.

Then there's the estrogen loss story on top of that. Heart disease is currently the number-one cause of death in postmenopausal women; in fact, more women die of heart disease than of lung cancer or breast cancer. Half of all North Americans who die from heart attacks each year are women.

One of the reasons for such high death rates from heart attacks among women is medical ignorance: most studies looking at heart disease excluded women, and that led to the myth that more men than women die of heart disease. The truth is, more men die of heart attacks before age 50, while more women die of heart attacks after age 50, as a direct result of estrogen loss. Moreover, women who have had oophorectomies (removal of the ovaries) prior to natural menopause increase their risk of a heart attack by *eight times*. But since more women work outside the home than ever before, a number of experts cite stress as a huge contributing factor to increased rates of heart disease in women.

Another problem is that women have different symptoms than men when it comes to heart disease, and so the "typical" warning signs we know about in men—angina, or chest pains—are often never present in women. In fact, chest pains in women are almost never related to heart disease. For women, the symptoms of heart disease, and even of an actual heart attack, can be much more vague, seemingly unrelated to heart problems. Signs of heart disease in women include some surprising symptoms; some are the same as in men, but some are completely different:

- Shortness of breath and/or fatigue
- Jaw pain (often masked by arthritis and joint pain)
- Pain in the back of the neck (often masked by arthritis or joint pain)
- Pain down the right or left arm
- Back pain (often masked by arthritis and joint pain)

- Sweating (also have your thyroid checked; this is a classic sign of an overactive thyroid gland; also test your blood sugar, as you may be low)
- Fainting
- Palpitations (ladies, again, have your thyroid checked, also a classic symptom of an overactive thyroid)
- Bloating (after menopause, this is a sign of coronary artery blockage)
- Heartburn, belching, or other gastrointestinal pain (this is often a sign of an actual heart attack in women)
- Chest "heaviness" between the breasts (this is how women experience "chest pain"; some describe it as a "sinking feeling" or burning sensation, an "aching, throbbing, or a squeezing sensation," a "hot poker stab in the chest," or "your heart jumping into your throat")
- Vomiting
- Confusion

Clearly, there are a lot of other causes for the symptoms on this list, but it's important for your doctor to explore heart disease as a possible cause, rather than dismissing it because your symptoms are not "male" (which your doctor may refer to as "typical").

Recovering from a Heart Attack

You can recover from a heart attack, but the extent of the damage caused by the attack greatly depends on how long the blood supply to the heart muscle was cut off. The longer the blood supply was cut off, the more damage you will have suffered. We all know that a heart attack is a major cause of death, but it can also leave you with varying degrees of disability depending upon the severity of the attack. For example, roughly half of all heart attack survivors will continue to have heart-related problems, such as reduced blood flow to the heart, called *ischemia*, and chest pains. You may also feel more fatigued and winded after normal activities when recovering from a heart attack. As a result, the lifestyle you once enjoyed will need to change: you may need to quit smoking, your diet will have to be restricted to one that's "heart smart," or you should find ways to reduce lifestyle stress and incorporate more activity into your routine. Successful recovery greatly depends on the severity of the attack and lifestyle changes you make after the episode. The same medical strategies designed to prevent a first heart attack can also be used to avoid recurrent episodes.

How Can I Prevent Cardiovascular Disease?

You can best prevent heart disease by cutting out the aggravating factors, such as smoking. Next, it's important that you get some insight into the causes of your stress and find ways to manage it. Then there's the boring stuff: eat well, stay active.

More invasive medical strategies involve heart surgery such as angioplasty and taking preventive medications.

Women and Stroke

Cardiovascular disease puts you at risk not just for a heart attack, but also for a "brain attack," or stroke, which occurs when a blood clot (a clog in your blood vessels) travels to your brain and stops the flow of blood and oxygen carried to the nerve cells in that area. When that happens, cells may die or vital functions controlled by the brain can be temporarily or permanently damaged. Bleeding or a rupture from the affected blood vessel can lead to a very serious situation, including death. About 80 percent of strokes are caused by the blockage of an artery in the neck or brain, known as an *ischemic stroke,* something that migraine sufferers can be prone to; the remainder are caused by a burst blood vessel in the brain that causes bleeding into or around the brain.

Since the 1960s, the death rate from strokes has dropped by 50 percent. This drop is largely due to public-awareness campaigns regarding diet and lifestyle modification (quitting smoking, eating low-fat foods, and exercising), as well as to the introduction of drugs that have helped people maintain normal blood pressure and cholesterol levels.

Strokes can be mild, moderate, severe, or fatal. Mild strokes may affect speech or movement for a short period of time only; many people recover from mild strokes without any permanent damage. Moderate or severe strokes may result in loss of speech, loss of memory, and paralysis; many people learn to speak again and learn to function with partial paralysis. How well a person recovers depends on how much damage was done.

A considerable amount of research points to stress as a major risk factor for stroke. Obviously you're tackling this problem if you're reading this book!

Signs of a Stroke

If you can recognize the key warning signs of a stroke, you can improve your chances of preventing a major stroke or reducing the severity of a stroke. Call 911 or get to Emergency if you *suddenly* notice one or more of the following symptoms:

- Weakness, numbness, and/or tingling in your face, arms, or legs, especially on one side of the body; this may last only a few moments.
- Loss of speech or difficulty understanding somebody else's speech; this may last only a short time.
- Confusion
- Severe headaches that feel different from any headache you've had before
- Feeling unsteady, falling a lot
- Trouble seeing in one or both eyes

If you have any of the signs of stroke above, it's important to get to the hospital as soon as possible. There are treatments that can reduce the severity of the damage caused by the stroke, making the difference between partial or severe disability and full recovery. For example, there are drugs that can dissolve clots, known as tissue-type plasminogen activators (TPAs), such as reteplase or streptokinase, which are proteins derived from bacteria. Plasminogen activators made from recombinant DNA technology are alteplase and anistreplase. Anticoagulant drugs, such as Coumadin, can dissolve clots as well.

More Severe PMS

While under stress, many women experience more severe premenstrual discomfort. Table 1.1 identifies all of the physical problems women experience as a result of stress, and cross-checks these problems against the premenstrual physical changes. Progesterone receptors do not function in the presence of adrenaline, the main stress hormone, which we also make when our blood sugar is low. This is huge news that may solve the PMS problems of millions of women. For more information on PMS see my book *Managing PMS Naturally: A sourcebook of Natural Solutions.*

TABLE 1.1   Stress or PMS?

Unique to Stress	Unique to PMS	Common to Stress and PMS
Dental and periodontal problems	Abdominal bloating (which may also cause weight gain)	Allergies and asthma
Herpes recurrences (especially in women)	Breast swelling and tenderness	Back pain
High blood pressure	Chills, shakiness, and dizziness	Changes in sex drive (either more or less)
High cholesterol	Clumsiness and poor coordination	Depression
Loss of appetite and weight loss	Constipation	Diarrhea
Premature aging	Eye problems	Emotional outbursts (rage, anger, crying, irritation—seen in recent reports on "air rage" and "desk rage")
	Hoarseness	Fatigue
	Increased appetite and weight gain	Gastrointestinal problems (digestive disorders, bowel problems, and so on)
	Nausea	Headaches
	Menopausal-like hot flashes	Heart pounding
	Seizures	Immune suppression (predisposing us to viruses, such as colds and flu; infections; autoimmune disorders, and cancer)
	Sensitivity to noise	Insomnia
	Sugar and salt cravings	Joint and muscle pain
		Skin problems and rashes

This chapter has looked at some of the most common stress-related physical health problems that women suffer. It is not exhaustive, however, and there are many health problems, ranging from herpes to skin rashes, that are not covered here. The main message is this: if you are experiencing physical health problems or strange symptoms while under stress, lowering your stress level could well be the key to regaining physical health.

2 THE EMOTIONAL SIGNS
OF A WOMAN'S STRESS

Which comes first, stress or the anxiety/panic/depression cycle to which most stressed-out women can succumb? When we're under stress, we may be irritable, sleep-deprived, or fatigued, all of which can make us feel things more intensely. But—and this is a big but—it's also accurate to say that when we're feeling a lot of emotions, we can become stressed. Emotional upset takes a real, calculable, physical toll on our bodies. The lines between stress and powerful emotions blur; they are interconnected. Not only are they hard to separate, but I wonder if they're even worth separating. The emotional signs of stress are anxiety, panic, and depression. All three problems come with their own set of physical and emotional sensations, which this chapter will explore.

Anxiety and Panic

In late August 2001, a few of my close female friends confided to me that they had been feeling quite anxious lately, to the point where they feared they were suffering from some sort of anxiety disorder. The general feeling among these women was one of impending doom, an unexplained fear that bordered on panic. The friends with children felt tremendous anxiety about the possibility that harm would come to their children. I asked each of them about their lives: were they under any unusual stress; how were their love lives going, etc. They each reported that nothing explained this new anxiety. It did not make sense. Something had to be wrong. Then the horror of September 11, 2001, occurred, and all of the women in this circle felt that their unfounded anxiety was somehow linked to that event. They believed they had sensed that "something" was in the air.

In a broader context, this is known as *ecofeminism,* a field of study that examines the connection between women and nature, as well as women's deeper connections with the environment surrounding them. In lay terms, it's a field that looks at women as creatures "in tune with their world" in a way that men are not. Women frequently sense dangers in their natural or socio-political environment, dangers that may be laughed off or trivialized by family members, colleagues, or friends.

In the early 1930s, American female journalist Sigrid Schultz gained access to Hitler as the Nazis were rising to power. She travelled to Denmark to wire stories to the *Chicago Tribune,* under the pseudonym John Dickson, warning of the dangers of Hitler and the Nazi party, and she accurately predicted what would happen if Germany gained too much power, which countries it would invade, and which countries would take its side. She was the first to write of the threat the Nazis posed to world peace and the first to report on the concentration camps. No other American had such close access to the Nazis. In the 1930s other journalists portrayed Hitler as a minor power who did not pose a threat. Schultz's warnings went unnoticed by the U.S. government. (Even though all of her predictions came true, she is scarcely mentioned in the history books.)

Rachel Carson, in 1962, wrote *Silent Spring,* a plea to industry to stop using pesticides. She reasoned that since these chemicals were killing fish and pond life in her backyard, soon they would be killing us. Carson was denounced as a heretic for daring to suggest that chemicals were destroying people's health, but as if in a Greek tragedy, she herself died from breast cancer at a younger than average age. (I've written about environmental causes of breast cancer in other books.)

A more modern example of ecofeminism is women's early clarion call about the Taliban regime's treatment of Afghan women. The petitions circulated by women's groups and then sent to democratic leaders, pleading that democracy was in danger if women were allowed to be treated in such a manner, went largely ignored until September 11, 2001. The film *Behind the Veil* would never have been shown on mainstream television networks had the attacks in New York and Washington not occurred. It is not uncommon for women to report feelings of anxiety and panic to their doctors, only to be told that their anxieties are unfounded, their fears exaggerated, when, in fact, there indeed has been something "in the air."

For many women, the issue of trust is the source of much anxiety. In the film *Mansfield Park,* the heroine has an opportunity to marry a fine, handsome young man who seems to be what every woman wants. But she refuses his affections because she simply does not trust him, even though she cannot offer the reason why.

> A couple of years ago I began to date a very nice guy who seemed genuinely interested in me and who appeared to be aggressively pursuing me. He called frequently, and we went out about half a dozen times before things got physical. I had told him on past dates that I was getting over another relationship and needed time. I was also unsure about whether I was even attracted to him and didn't know if the right chemistry would be there. When he kissed me, I decided to "go with the flow." I was pleasantly surprised by how much chemistry was there, and felt very happy that it was there for me, since all the other elements—intelligence, humour, and so on—were there as well. Things took their natural course and we wound up making love. Afterwards, he held me, said all the right things—including "Let's just take it slow"—and left about 3:00 a.m. because he needed to be at work early and wanted to get home. It all sounded reasonable. He called me the next day (Thursday) and said he was going away for the weekend. On Monday afternoon, when I didn't hear from him, I started to become very anxious and panicky—to the point where I was paralyzed with fear and went to bed. I called one of my close friends and told her I was having a bad moment and that something was wrong. The fear was familiar—a fear that I would be left and abandoned, which was a pattern in my relationships. My girlfriend told me that I was just worrying for nothing: "If things went as well as you say they did, there's no reason for him not to call you again. He probably wants to take it slow and not rush things—just like he told you." I finally bit the bullet and called him; he had apparently just returned late that morning from his weekend. He suggested we get together, and I called my girlfriend back and told her that she was right. Otherwise, why would he want to see me? When we got together, we spent about an hour chatting about trivial matters. Then he told me that he felt no chemistry and didn't want to see me again. I was shocked, but somehow comforted that my earlier anxiety was warranted. Now when I feel that anxious feeling with a man, I know he is not to be trusted.

Subtle changes in behaviour are often sensed unconsciously, and anxiety and panic may be our first signs that there is something truly unsettling about a person or situation. Women can also detect subtle changes in their work environments, often sensing when their jobs are in peril. Frequently, there is no way to prove that what we are feeling makes any sense. Sometimes women need only to look at their lives to understand why they are suffering from anxiety and/or panic (the two usually go together—like "love and marriage" or "horse and carriage"). Chapter 4 takes a closer look at many causes of anxiety and panic—family life and relationships chiefly. Too many responsibilities, not feeling trust or safe in a relationship, lacking the security to express yourself in troubled family relationships—all these cause anxiety and panic.

Chapter 5, which looks at women in the workplace, covers many other common sources of anxiety and panic. When we are compromised in our jobs or asked to do things that go against our own moral centre, we can experience tremendous anxiety and panic.

> After our hospital suffered severe nursing shortages, I was moved from the oncology floor to the neonatal floor, where many premature babies are kept on life-support. Many times, I had to assist in keeping babies—who were clearly going to die—alive with invasive procedures that I thought were just plain wrong. I kept feeling that we were needlessly torturing these poor little helpless beings who were technically not even viable human lives (because they could not survive outside the womb yet). I was never asked for my opinion and even if I had been, since nurses have no voice in the hospital system, I felt that expressing my opinion would just put my job in jeopardy for nothing. I began to suffer from terrible anxiety and panic attacks when I was off-duty. It got to the point where I couldn't work in that environment. Now I work as a private nurse for a home-care agency.

Generalized Anxiety Disorder

When it comes to stress-related anxiety, we are talking about something known as *generalized anxiety disorder* (GAD). GAD is characterized by extreme worry about things that are unlikely to happen. You may worry about whether your child is safe or whether your partner is going to get into a car accident on the way home. You may begin to worry about health problems. Your worries begin to be persistent and interfere with your normal functioning. Always there is a sense of dread, a constant "fretting," restlessness, and uneasiness about your personal security or safety. You may also suffer from physical symptoms:

- Clenched teeth or jaw
- Tightened muscles
- Holding your breath
- Sleeping problems
- Racing heartbeat
- Breathing difficulties
- Chest pain
- Hyperventilation

Anxiety can also accompany depression, which I discuss further on.

Anxiety versus Normal Worry

It's normal to worry about a lot of things. Worry crosses over into "anxiety" when the worry persists after the problem you worried about has ended or been resolved. Normally, after a problem has been resolved, a sense of calm or even satisfaction follows. For example, if you found a lump in your breast, you would naturally be anxious about it until you had it evaluated. When you are told by your doctor that the lump is benign and not cancerous, it would be natural at this point for you to feel relief. When you suffer from anxiety, you don't get the relief. You begin to think: What if the doctor made a mistake? What if I'm not fine? This is anxiety.

Or, let's say you have a job performance review coming up. It would be natural for you to worry about it or be anxious beforehand, but if the review goes well, you should feel relief. If, however, you begin to worry about whether you "should have" said what you did or whether you "should have" said things you didn't say, and then begin to wonder how secure your job really is, you may be suffering from anxiety.

In other words, if you're always worrying about *something*, you may benefit from counselling or therapy. Being in a constant state of worry disrupts your life and prevents you from functioning normally.

Anxiety in the Face of Terrorism

Today, in light of the world events as of this writing, more than two-thirds of Canadians in recent polls report that they are suffering from anxiety. People are worried about flying, opening the mail, working in high-rise buildings. It's not that there aren't good reasons for these worries, but we just can't live this way for too long—it takes too much of a toll on our minds and bodies. We have to find ways to live in the world knowing that we are vulnerable to danger. This is how humans have survived since time began.

As a cancer survivor, I have started to think of terrorism as a diagnosis of "global cancer." When someone is first diagnosed with cancer, it doesn't mean that the cancer wasn't there for a long time; it just means that the person is now *aware* of the cancer. Similarly, terrorists have been around for a long time (they've been a recognized reality in many countries for decades); what's changed in North America is that now we are *aware* of them in our midst. The danger has always been there; now we just know about it for sure. People went on with their lives all through the Cold War under the constant threat of nuclear annihilation. World danger is nothing new. There will always be misery and suffering, danger and vulnerability. This is what human life is about: being aware of our mortality and vulnerability.

These days, many people are cancelling travel plans that involve airplanes. This can be looked upon as a reasonable precaution in uncertain times. Taking trains, cars, or buses to various destinations are alternatives that make sense for many people; they're still carrying on with their lives and plans, but they're making some changes to accommodate some of their worries. Anxiety becomes a problem when we start to avoid life. Being afraid to go outside at all, fearing danger, is not a healthy reaction. When our fear is so overwhelming and intense that it disrupts our lives, we have a problem.

The causes of anxiety for women are usually garden-variety socio-economic problems. Problems involving jobs, finances, relationships, and health are all common reasons for anxiety. But when you're under increased stress, normal worries can cross over into anxiety and low-level anxiety can also intensify or heighten.

When anxiety appears suddenly, too many normal socio-economic stressors may be happening all at once. For example, there may be a series of deaths in the family. Perhaps you have just lost your job and then discover you have cancer. Your mother may have just had a stroke, and then you find out that you owe thousands of dollars in taxes because of some computer glitch. One friend of mine had a year from hell: first, her newborn nephew was diagnosed with a rare cancer (he recovered after many "touch and go" treatments); then her father died suddenly from complications after a common surgical procedure; then her mother was diagnosed with cancer (she is now recovering and doing just fine).

Alternatively, sudden anxiety may be the result of completely new changes in your life:

- Were you a victim of crime? Or do old traumas still bother you? In this case, your feelings of anxiety may be part of what's now called *post-traumatic stress disorder*. This term has come to replace "shell shock" and was first used to describe the trauma-related anxiety that Vietnam war veterans suffered years after their war experiences. The traumatic experience may have been limited to one event, such as a rape or assault, accident, or fire, or it may have been prolonged, such as years of enduring sexual abuse, surviving a concentration camp or war, or being a victim of stalking.

- Have you begun to take any new medications or substances? Anxiety can be triggered by many medications as well as by illegal substances, such as cocaine. (See Chapter 3.)

- Have you moved or changed jobs?

- Are you grieving over the loss of a loved one or relationship? (See Chapter 7.)

When you suffer from anxiety, you may also suffer from panic attacks. In the Introduction to this book, I described an extreme panic attack that I had. A panic attack is so named because it is an "attack"—it comes on suddenly without warning. Because there is no warning, once you've had one panic attack, you can easily begin to worry about when the next one might strike. The fear of reliving a panic attack in public can become so overwhelming that you may be afraid to leave your house. This is known as *agoraphobia*: the fear of going outside. When you are at home, you're in a safe place for a panic attack, but when you're in a public place (as I was), the panic is heightened, and so, too, can be the symptoms of the attack.

The symptoms of a panic attack are brought on by a rush of adrenaline—a stress hormone that gets triggered in a fight-or-flight response. Diabetics who suffer from episodes of low blood sugar have the same response, as adrenaline gets pumped out when blood sugar is low. If you're suffering from anxiety, you often don't eat well, so panic attacks can be exacerbated by low blood sugar.

When the adrenaline pumps out, your heart rate accelerates—this often feels not like a palpitation, but more like a "fluttery" heartbeat; it can also feel racing, pounding, or skipping. This is accompanied by a cold sweat or excessive sweating, chills or flushes (a.k.a. cold or hot flashes), and possibly tingling or numbness in parts of your body. What happens next depends on what's going on in your life: Some people begin to feel *vertigo* symptoms: extreme dizziness, lightheadedness, shakiness, nausea, and other stomach problems. Other people begin to feel *choking* symptoms: rapid breathing or hyperventilating, shortness of breath, a choking or smothering sensation, a lump in the throat, and chest pain, pressure, or discomfort. As one therapist put it to me, people who feel that their world is collapsing tend to have "vertigo-like" panic attacks, as their symptoms mirror how they feel; while people who feel they have too much responsibility or weight on their shoulders tend to have "choking-like" panic attacks, as their symptoms mirror how they feel, too.

Whether the symptoms are of the vertigo or choking variety, there is also a feeling of unreality about panic attacks; you may feel you are caught in a bad dream or that you are detached from your body and are having distorted perceptions. A fear of losing control or embarrassing yourself, a sense of impending doom, or a fear of dying may also be part of the experience. You may also pass out. When you begin to notice panic attack symptoms, you may start to panic even more because the situation is so frightening and jarring.

Roughly 2 percent of North Americans aged 18 to 54 suffer from panic attacks each year, and attacks occur twice as often in women as in men. Although chronic panic attacks often occur before age 24, many people suffer their first attack in their 30s and 40s while under extreme stress.

Managing Anxiety and Panic

Talk therapy is an excellent way to manage anxiety and panic. Finding a good therapist can be challenging (see pages 70–82 for suggestions on finding good counselling). Although it's common for women to be tossed a prescription for antidepressants or tranquilizers by family doctors or psychiatrists, the research on treatment shows that talk therapy—particularly cognitive behavioural therapy (see page 78)—is often the best way to manage anxiety and panic. When someone validates what you're feeling and gives you some real, hands-on life-management skills as an anchor, it's amazing how much better you feel. Antidepressants, anti-anxiety agents, and drugs that slow your heart down and calm you while you're in the throes of a panic attack have a role in treatment, too, but all reasonable mental health practitioners believe in this adage: Start low, go slow. You should always start with the least invasive therapy before moving on to something that could have side-effects.

Next time you're in the throes of a panic attack, here are three natural things to try (you should always carry these remedies with you):

1. Breathe into a paper bag. This will slow down your heart naturally, since you are breathing in more carbon dioxide.

2. Take the homeopathic Rescue Remedy for panic and anxiety discussed in Chapter 10. These are drops that you take orally when you feel the panic beginning.

3. Take the essential oil "orange." This calms the heart. When you feel the panic coming on, apply the oil to the nape of your neck, the thymus gland at the front of your neck, and the soles of your feet. The oil should penetrate quickly and help calm you.

A Word about Health Anxiety

Health anxiety is an anxiety/panic that is confined to your health. People who suffer from health anxiety are usually healthy, but they are overly sensitive to bodily sensations and quickly jump from "What's this itch?" to the belief they are dying from some horrible disease. People with health anxiety may go from doctor to doctor looking for "answers" to their symptoms; they become more and more frustrated when they're told that there's nothing wrong. The symptoms of panic and anxiety, indeed, are responsible for many of the physical symptoms that plague people with health anxiety: numbness, tingling, stomach trouble, headaches, twitching, odd sensations, flushes, and heart palpitations. These sufferers may also spend hours on the Internet looking up rare diseases (a.k.a. cyberchondria), believing they are dying from one thing on Monday and another thing on Friday. Common beliefs are that they are dying of multiple sclerosis, cancer, ALS, or a brain tumour. People who suffer from health anxiety frequently have OCD, or obsessive compulsive disorder, where the obsessions are focused on the body. If you believe you suffer from health anxiety, a good website to visit is **www.healthanxiety.com**.

Stress-Related Depression

It's important to understand that depression is a vast topic and that there are many different types of depression. In the context of stress-related depression, the type of depression that is triggered is called *unipolar depression,* a depression characterized by one low mood. This is distinct from *bipolar depression,* a mood disorder in which there are two moods: one high and one low. Most cases of unipolar depression are caused by life circumstances and/or situations. For this reason, mental health experts use the term *situational depression* to describe most cases of mild, moderate, or even severe unipolar depression. Among other things, situational depression can mean that your depression has been triggered by a life event. Examples of a life event include:

- Illness
- Loss of a loved one (the relationship may have ended or a loved one may have died)
- Major life change
- Job loss or change
- Moving

Situational depression may also have been triggered by the *absence* of change in your life, meaning that you are living in a state of continuous struggle, unhappiness, or stress and that there's no light at the end of the tunnel. Examples of states of continuous struggle include

- Chronic illness

- Unhealthy relationships

- Poverty and/or economic worries

- Job stress

- Body-image problems, such as feeling fat or unattractive

A third kind of situational depression is one triggered by an absence of resolution regarding past traumas and abuses you suffered as a child or younger adult. Examples of past traumas include:

- Sexual abuse

- Incest

- Violence

- Rape

- Emotional abuse

One out of five people in Canada can expect to suffer from depression. That's a lot, considering that a Canadian's lifetime risk of asthma is only 1 in 20. At least twice as many women suffer from depression as men, but statistics from the National Population Health Survey show even higher numbers for women. For example, from 1994 through 1997, 72 percent of reported depressive episodes involved women. There are some reasons for this. Women in their 20s and 30s, for example, are at risk for postpartum depression because of a lack of social supports for women with newborns. This issue is discussed further in Chapter 4. Generally, social conditions for women are more difficult than they are for men, and women tend to seek help more often than men do. Since women live longer than men, in their later years more women than men grieve over the loss of a spouse or feel isolated as a result of the aging process.

Sadness versus Depression

The million-dollar question is this: Are you depressed or "just sad"? Everyone experiences sadness, bad days, and bad moods. Feeling sad is not the same thing as depression. So the first order of business is to define what normal sadness is and understand how it is distinct from depression.

What exactly is sadness? "Sadness," per se, can be defined as mental anguish or suffering in the absence of any physical pain, the kind of feeling experienced when a loved one dies. A mother watching her child suffer, for example, is not in any physical pain, but she still suffers and experiences sadness. When we are sad, we express our emotions by crying, talking, or thinking continuously about our sorrow. We may find it difficult to sleep or concentrate, and we may be unable to eat. Sadness is characterized by sad *feelings*; it is the opposite of numbness—the main feature of depression.

A problem for many people in affluent cultures is that their sadness isn't triggered by anything obvious. For example, we can become sad when we realize that our life circumstances or situations are not improving. Stagnating, "being in a rut," and finding that life is getting worse rather than better are conditions that lead to sadness and suffering. As human beings, we are driven toward self-actualization once our basic needs (safety, food, shelter, love) are looked after. But when our life circumstances stymie self-actualization or spiritual growth, we suffer and feel sad. The longing for material possessions, money, or an intimate relationship is often just an expression of longing for self-realization. Later in life, many of us begin to question our attachments to material possessions and power; we begin to see the difference between real needs (i.e., love, friendship, respect) and artificial needs (i.e., money, power, prestige).

For those of us who are content with things as they are, sadness and suffering can develop when a life event of some kind threatens the status quo, our identity or selfhood, or our quality of life. The threat can be almost anything, of course, ranging from physical illness (such as breast cancer) to financial hardship.

The main thing to remember about sadness versus depression is this: sadness *lifts*, depression *persists*. That's how you can determine whether you're just feeling sad or are actually depressed. Feelings of sadness and grief are common and normal reactions to an infinite variety of circumstances. And, again, the symptoms of sadness often mirror those of depression: you're crying; you can't sleep; you can't eat. But eventually, as time passes and you find yourself going back to your routine, the sadness *lifts*. While you may still be sad or grieving, you can also enjoy your life and put your sad thoughts on the back burner. That's not to say that the problem has disappeared, but you will be able to cope with the right support. You may need to talk about your problem or life event to friends or family, but every day gets easier. You can get out of bed and have appreciation for something in life, whether it's a nice day, a funny movie, or a good dessert. When you're depressed, nothing lifts. Life gets greyer, bleaker, and more difficult until you begin to feel numb, and what you once found pleasurable no longer interests you. Your ability to function will *decrease* with each passing day when you're depressed; your ability to function will *increase* with each passing day when you're just sad about something. But the trigger—the event that has caused you to be sad or depressed—is always real, understandable, and legitimate. Never forget that.

The tricky thing about the sadness-versus-depression question is that what triggered your sadness can also trigger a depression. Again, if the symptoms persist rather than lift, you may need some help. When sadness lifts, you can relate to the song lyric "I can see clearly now, the rain is gone." When depression persists, you are in that "dark cloud that has you blind." I don't mean to be glib, but sometimes songs really do say it best.

Signs of Depression

Depression is clinically known as a *mood disorder*. It's impossible to define what a "normal mood" is, since we all have such complex personalities and exhibit different moods throughout a given week or even a given day. But it's not impossible for *you* to define what a normal mood is for *you*. You know how you feel when you're functional: you're eating, sleeping, and interacting with friends and family; you're productive, active, and generally interested in the daily goings-on in life. Well, depression is the feeling that for a long period of time you haven't had the ability to function or, even if you appear to the outside world to be functioning at a reasonable level, you haven't had any *interest* in participating in life.

One bad day, or even a bad week (which will usually include moments when you can take pleasure in something), from time to time, is not necessarily a sign that you're depressed. Feeling you've lost the ability to function as you *normally* do, all day, every day, for a period of at least two weeks may be a sign that you're depressed.

> I was in the midst of a very stressful ad campaign and needed to work up new copy for a presentation the next day. Normally, I would take my laptop home, take a bath, and the "creative" would just come. I was considered to be the creative genius at my agency. I had been feeling sort of all over the place and wasn't really myself, but I didn't realize how bad it was until I couldn't clear my head when I was soaking in my tub. That night, I took six baths, hoping that the juices would come back. At 2:00 a.m., when I still had nothing, I started to get out of the tub. It was then I felt my heart racing and sinking all at once. I couldn't breathe, so I just sat down and tried to calm myself by splashing cold water on my face from the tub faucet. I called a freelancer I knew, left an urgent message, and subbed out the project, paying him out of my own pocket. Things just got worse at work, and I felt as though I had lost the ability to think. In the end, everything was a mess and I left my job. Then I left my boyfriend. Then I left my apartment. Everyone said I had burnout. The truth is, I was tired of the constant stress of that job, the "no-wheresville" of my commitment-phobic, toxic boyfriend, and my mouse-infested apartment.

The symptoms of depression can vary from person to person, but can include some or all of the following:

- Feelings of sadness and/or emptiness
- Difficulty sleeping (usually waking up frequently in the middle of the night)
- Loss of energy and feelings of fatigue and lethargy
- Change in appetite (usually a loss of appetite)
- Difficulty thinking, concentrating, or making decisions
- Loss of interest in formerly pleasurable activities, including sex
- Anxiety or panic attacks (see page 57)
- Obsessing over negative experiences or thoughts
- Feeling guilty, worthless, hopeless, or helpless
- Feeling restless and irritable
- Thinking about death or suicide

When You Can't Sleep

The typical sleep pattern of a depressed person is to go to bed at their normal time only to wake up around 2:00 a.m. and be unable get back to sleep. Endless hours are spent watching infomercials to pass the time, or simply tossing and turning, usually obsessing over negative experiences or thoughts. Lack of sleep affects our ability to function and leads to increased irritability, lack of energy, and fatigue. Insomnia, by itself, is not a sign of depression, but if depression is seen as a package of symptoms, the inability to fall or stay asleep can aggravate all the other symptoms. In other cases, people who are depressed will oversleep, requiring 10 to 12 hours of sleep every night.

When You Can't Think Clearly

Another debilitating feature of depression is finding that you simply can't concentrate or think clearly. You feel scattered, disorganized, and unable to prioritize. This usually hits hardest in the workplace or a centre of learning, and it can severely impair your performance. You may miss important deadlines or important meetings, or find that you can't focus when you do go to meetings. When you can't think clearly, you can be overwhelmed with feelings of helplessness or hopelessness. "I can't even perform a simple task such as X anymore" may dominate your thoughts as you become more disillusioned with your dwindling productivity.

Anhedonia: When Nothing Gives You Pleasure

One of the most telling signs of depression is a loss of interest in activities that used to excite you, enthuse you, or give you pleasure. This is known as *anhedonia*, derived from the word "hedonism" ("the philosophy of pleasure"). A hedonist is a person who indulges her every pleasure without considering (or caring about) the consequences. Anhedonia simply means "no pleasure."

Different people have different ways of expressing anhedonia. You might tell your friends, for example, that you have no desire to do X or Y; you can't get motivated; or X or Y just doesn't hold your interest or attention. You may also notice that the sense of satisfaction from a job well done is simply gone; this is particularly debilitating in the workplace or in a place of learning. For example, artists (photographers, painters, writers, etc.) may find that the passion has gone out of their work.

Many of the other symptoms of depression also hinge on loss of pleasure. One of the reasons weight loss is so common in depression (typically, people may notice as much as a 10-pound drop in their weight) is that food no longer gives pleasure and/or cooking no longer gives pleasure. The sense of satisfaction we get from having a clean home or clean kitchen may also disappear. Therefore, the prospect of having to clean up our kitchens in order to prepare food may seem too taxing, contributing to a lack of interest in food.

Of course, gaining weight is also not unusual: 10 pounds in the opposite direction can occur, too. This is often due to poor nutrition: when we're depressed, we're not motivated to prepare or eat well-balanced meals, and so we fill up on snack foods or high-calorie, low-nutrient foods. Weight gain may also come from a loss of interest in physical activities; we may avoid exercising, sports, or the dozen other things that keep us active when we're feeling "ourselves."

A loss of interest in sex aggravates matters if we are in a sexual relationship with someone. Again, the decreased desire for sex stems from general anhedonia.

Women who suffer from depression also report feelings of self-blame or self-hatred as well as physical symptoms such as headaches and gastrointestinal problems.

What Causes Depression?

Since most episodes of depression are triggered by life events or circumstances, the causes of depression are different for everyone. In a very general way, the direct answer to the question "Who gets depressed?" is this: people living in difficult circumstances. Understanding what's "difficult" is akin to understanding pain thresholds. What one woman finds difficult, another may not.

What we also know is that depression—or at least the *diagnosis* of depression—is on the rise. One should note that when there is awareness of and active screening for a particular condition, there is a rise in incidence (in this case, active screening is done through diagnostic criteria listed in the DSM IV, which stands *for Diagnostic and Statistical Manual of Mental Disorders,* 4th edition, an often-criticized "recipe book" on psychiatric symptoms put out by the American Psychiatric Association). In other words, when you're looking for something, you'll find it. But of course, *not* looking for something doesn't mean it isn't there. The question remains: is it better to seek out depression and treat it, ending unnecessary suffering? Many health-care practitioners would answer, "Yes!"

U.S. statistics show that people born after 1940 suffer from depression and other mood disorders more than those born before that time. But that says much more about the social structure that has emerged since 1940 than it does about people— specifically, women—and depression. There is no proof, however, that more women are depressed today than were depressed during, say, the Great Depression. That's because no one looked into how many women were depressed during that time; if someone had, it is likely she or he would have found rather high numbers of depressed women, given the lot of women at that time and the economic misery of the period.

Here's where the brain chemistry story comes in. Brain chemistry is *altered* in depressed people, but this physical alteration only occurs *after* a stressor has already thrown them into a depression. Brain chemistry doesn't just change spontaneously, in the *absence* of an environmental trigger (see Chapter 1 for discussion about environ- mental triggers).

The Genetic Link

With so many likely triggers to depression, it's logical to ask: "Why isn't everyone depressed? Why only me?" Some researchers believe that some people have a *genetic predisposition* to depression. For example, let's say you had a genetic predisposition to lung cancer. If you never smoked, chances are you wouldn't develop lung cancer. But if you smoked, you could potentially trip the lung cancer switch. On the other hand, if you didn't have a genetic predisposition to lung cancer, you could smoke a pack of cigarettes until you were 90 and still never develop lung cancer. It works the same way with biological depressive illnesses. The "cigarettes" in this case are difficult life circumstances, unforeseen stresses and tragedies, and other random acts of misfortune. Some of these circumstances we can control; others are *beyond* our control, requiring us to tap into inner strengths, belief systems, and coping skills.

There are many who criticize genetic research into depression. While no specific gene has yet been found for biological depressive illnesses, the hunt is definitely on, and it is a potentially dangerous hunt. Although it's clear to researchers that depression has many causes and that no one gene will likely be found to "cause" various kinds of depression, the worry is that once certain genes are even linked to depression, there may be a tendency to lose sight of the significance of environmental triggers. In other words, instead of, say, putting an emphasis on the need to enact legislation to protect women from domestic violence—a major trigger for depression—more emphasis will be placed on altering the battered woman's brain chemistry with drugs.

Furthermore, who will try to exert some control with respect to the potential social harms associated with "depression genes"? What if we find that some minority or ethnic groups have more depression genes than other groups? This could potentially blacklist these groups from certain kinds of jobs, for example. What if women are offered a prenatal test for depression genes and are given the opportunity to terminate pregnancies for fetuses that test positive? Would that be a good thing? These are unanswerable, and even unasked, questions at this stage. But the simple fact remains that life is difficult and some people have less support and poorer coping skills—and more to cope with—than others.

Managing Depression

When your depression is stress-related, talk therapy is the first logical step. (See the section "Finding Someone to Talk To," page 70.) Talk therapy can be combined with herbal mood lifters and antidepressant medications, but, again, consider the "Start low, go slow" adage when you're seeking treatment for depression.

Herbal Remedies

In 1997 the American Psychiatric Association stated that the herb St. John's wort could be used as a first-line treatment for mild to moderate depression. The herb is named after St. John, the patron saint of nurses, while "wort" is simply Old English for "plant." It is essentially the "nurse's plant." St. John's wort can apparently also work in many people as a prescription antidepressant because it relieves stress. It is also known, therefore, to relieve other stress-related problems, including gastrointestinal ailments.

St. John's wort has been used successfully for years throughout Europe. Several studies show that it can do the same job as antidepressants without as many side-effects (see Chapter 10 for a more detailed description of this herb).

Antidepressants

Antidepressants work on your brain chemistry. They have side-effects and are over-prescribed to women for depression, PMS, anxiety, and normal mood responses to difficult circumstances. Antidepressants have a legitimate role, but they should be reserved for severe cases of depression, where possible.

There are several types of prescription antidepressants, including heterocyclics, monamine oxidase inhibitors (MOIs), and selective serotonin reuptake inhibitors (SSRIs). A subtype of SSRIs, called MSRI (mixed serotonin reuptake inhibitors), is also popular and includes serotonin-norephinephrine reuptake inhibitors (SNRIs). For more information, consult my book *Women and Depression*.

Support Groups

The *sharing approach* has been shown to be highly beneficial, particularly in cases where women share difficult circumstances or problems. Professionals who provide counselling for women report that the support that women receive from other women helps them gain the confidence they need to deal with their problems.

This isn't just true for depression. Several studies have shown the value of support groups and support systems in treating many physical diseases, including cancer. One study found that women with end-stage breast cancer who joined a support group actually lived longer than women who did not. And women who share common conditions, such as infertility, AIDS, pregnancy loss, and so on, find support groups enormously helpful.

Since depression has so many causes, support groups for depressed women are not as useful as support groups for, say, women who are living with violence or women who are battling obesity. In other words, succeeding in finding or establishing a group of women who share your circumstances is the key to finding good support. Otherwise, you may wind up in a group where your particular circumstances are not understood at all. For example, if you are going through a divorce, someone coping with cancer may find your circumstances not reason enough for you to feel depressed.

Or, someone with AIDS may find it unreasonable for someone with a treatable cancer to have feelings of depression. And so on.

Community and cultural norms are also significant factors in the search for the right support group. For example, white women may cope differently with depression than black or Hispanic women. East Indian women may cope differently than Asian women, while African-American women may cope differently than Caribbean or Somali women.

Where do you look for support? If you're struggling to make ends meet, for example, and want to discuss your problems with others with your predicament, you won't likely find an ad in the paper inviting "All Poor Women" to a support group. But if you live in a poor community, you might find support by signing up for community-based programs, ranging from crafts groups to yoga. In fact, community-outreach workers use classes in arts, crafts, fitness, computer, and so on, as a means to attract women within the community who could benefit from support. What often takes place in community-based programs is a great deal of talking and sharing during, prior to, and after the activity. These are places where you make friends, find someone you can talk to, and, most importantly, find that you're not alone in your situation. Community programs are a way for women to say to their abusive husbands: "Back in an hour; I'm going to my yoga class," instead of: "I'm going to talk about what a bastard you are to a bunch of other women living with bastards!"

The old joke about women going to the bathroom "in twos" is quite accurate; women go together to the bathroom because it's a place where they can *talk*. Women need other women to talk to. This is how we've been coping with the hardships of life for centuries. One study found that women have an average of about four to six close friendships with other women; men average zero to one close friendships with another male.

What Women Talk About

When women talk informally to try to put their feelings into perspective, these are some of the things they talk about:

- **Sexism.** In case you haven't noticed, we live in a sexist society where men still enjoy more privileges than women. Ask other women how they feel about that. Your conversation won't change the world, but your feelings about the world might be validated. And that feels good.

- **Powerlessness.** You know what? You feel powerless because you're set up to feel powerless—by those in power! Most women have very little power in their workplace, home, community, and so forth. So it's no wonder you feel inadequate. Talking about this may help you find a perspective that actually empowers you. By the way, this is not to say that there are no powerful women in the world; it's just that they are few and far between. And there are plenty of women in power who feel powerless, too.

- **Ambivalence over Assertiveness.** I know it's the 21st century, but women in many cultures are still being taught to be docile and passive in a world that is aggressive and harsh. Again, talking about the need to be more assertive won't necessarily change you into a go-getter, but it will probably help you realize that you're not the only one out there who has been taught to feel that aggressiveness and assertiveness are unfeminine. Your reluctance to assert yourself is perfectly understandable, given the message you've been sent from birth: you do not have a voice, and if you speak, negative consequences will follow.

- **Absurd Standards of Beauty.** Spend an afternoon with a fashion photographer and makeup artist, and they'll tell you a few things. What you see in the magazines is fiction and fantasy, created with the use of heavy makeup, carefully arranged lighting, and computer-aided touch-ups. The real-life fashion model might actually have made herself vomit prior to the photo shoot (she can't fool the makeup artist, who can smell the vomit while working on her). Is that beautiful? Talk about *that* with other women! One makeup artist put it best when he told me: "I can't even watch television or read a magazine anymore because I know how ugly this business is and how desperate the women are who participate in this sham. We [makeup artists and photographers] spend hours distorting these women and dare call it 'beauty.'" Since it is the Caucasian face that is objectified and held up as the global standard of beauty, what are you supposed to do if you're not Caucasian? Does this standard of beauty make sense to you? And when 17-year-old girls are objectified and held up as an ideal that a 35-year-old woman should strive for, isn't that *insane*? Tall women (models must be at least five feet nine inches to get work) are taller than the average Caucasian woman, so if you're of average height for a Caucasian, you're not considered beautiful enough for the Western standard. But of course, most women on the planet are not Caucasian. Asian women, for example, are on average shorter than the average Caucasian woman. Again, our beauty standards verge on lunacy.

The point to seeking comfort in validation is not to confirm your suspicions that life is horrible and hopeless; rather it's to gain the sense that you're not the only one who feels that life is a struggle. This should give you the courage to move forward and make some changes (or at least make some friends who have common concerns) rather than shrink in a corner feeling you're the only one with your problem.

Family Support

Depression changes spousal/partner relationships as well as other family relationships. When you're going through a depression, knowing that things won't fall apart can be the source of greatest comfort. Unfortunately, too many women are treated to "family harassment" in the sense that they are not given the space to go through their depression. Being continuously told to "Snap out of it," "Get out of the house," "Go for a walk," or "What you need is a nice big cup of tea" isn't what family support is about. There are things family members can do that are supportive, things that will let you know that you are allowed to go through what you *are* going through.

Tips for Your Family and Friends

Family or friends may need some guidance on how to help. Here are some examples of what they can do for you.

1. They should become the homemaker without asking. You may have trouble asking for help and may worry about how everything will get done; this only adds to your burden, so it's important for family and friends to offer unsolicited help. When family or friends look after as many of the meals, chores, and so on as they can, it takes pressure off you.

2. If you want a family member or friend to go to a support group or counselling with you, they should agree to go. This says: "I want to understand what's going on with you."

3. Friends and family should check *in* with you rather than check *up*. Asking how you're feeling, how your kids are faring, and so on is fine and supportive, but badgering you with unwanted opinions or advice or asking, "What did you *do* today?" in a judgmental tone is *not* fine or supportive.

4. Those close to you must give you the feeling that you are "allowed" to set the pace of your day. When family members try to force you to go on an outing, eat, or do anything you don't feel like doing, it just puts more pressure on you and emphasizes your inability to function or cope.

5. If you want to tell people about your depression or feelings, you should feel an underlying support from friends and family to do so. People have different ways of coping, and some choose to be open about their mood disorder. You shouldn't feel as though depression is a dirty secret that must be hidden from view.

Finding Someone to Talk To

How do you know when you need help for stress-related anxiety, panic, or depression? In my own case, I had to literally collapse before I recognized that I needed therapy. If you feel you need help, you should seek it—even if family members or friends discourage you from this course. It can become a daunting task, however, to figure out *who* you should seek out, and for this reason, many women simply do not find proper help. This section will help you navigate your way through the sea of talk therapists and styles of talk therapies that are available to you.

In Search of a Good Therapist

When you're looking for a therapist, you should focus on finding someone you can relate to, someone who is a "good fit." The pitfall you want to avoid is winding up with a therapist who is not helpful. Unhelpful therapy does not mean that your therapist is an unethical or poor therapist; it means that the style of therapy isn't suitable for you and/or that your therapist is not someone with whom you feel entirely comfortable. There can be many reasons for a poor fit, and they are often difficult to nail down. In other words, what one woman finds helpful therapy another woman may not. Therapists and styles of therapy are highly individual and so are their impacts.

Locating Names

Assuming you are seeking help on your own, where do you begin? There are two general routes: referral or "going shopping." If you have a good primary-care doctor (general practitioner, family practitioner, internist, or, in some cases, a gynecologist whom you see more regularly than a primary-care doctor), that doctor can refer you to a few different therapists who specialize in depression or mood disorders. You're more likely to be referred to a psychiatrist or psychologist in this case. If you like your referring doctor, chances are you'll like one of the therapists she or he refers you to.

Many women can't count on their primary-care physician for such referrals. In some cases, they may feel uncomfortable disclosing their wish to seek out counselling; in others, they may not have a primary-care doctor at all—or one they like. Thankfully, there are many other options available, such as the following:

The Employee Assistance Program.
This program is now offered by many workplaces. The employer prepays a group of therapists for X number of hours of therapy. You call a toll-free number that is kept

completely confidential, whereupon you have the option of seeing various licensed therapists on a short-term basis. Some therapists specialize in addiction or stress management, while others specialize in depression. The program is relatively risk-free in that if you don't like the therapist you see, you simply don't go back. And it hasn't cost you anything.

Community Family Services or Women's Health Clinics.
Several communities operate family and child services, or women's clinics, where you can call to book an appointment with a staff social worker who can help you. You may be able to drop in unannounced, but calling ahead of time is always best. These services are usually not free, but you will be charged according to your ability to pay.

Hospitals.
If you're feeling overwhelmed and know you must speak to someone immediately, you can go straight to a hospital and request a consultation with a mental health professional in that hospital. Mental health professionals who work in hospitals include psychiatrists, clinical psychologists, psychiatric nurses, and social workers. You can sign yourself in as a voluntary patient if there is room. In this case, the province or territory will cover your initial consultation and, possibly, further treatment. You can be treated as an outpatient, too; this is a popular alternative for many women. Hospitals usually won't admit you unless you're threatening suicide or have attempted suicide in the past. (And sometimes even under these circumstances, you may be sent home, thanks to hospital cutbacks.)

Crisis Lines.
If you're feeling overwhelmed and need to speak to somebody right away, calling one of the crisis telephone lines listed in the front of your White Pages is an option. A crisis counsellor can also refer you to other people or places for longer-term counselling.

The "Blue Book."
Most urban areas have a community information services book or, at least, a list of community services phone numbers. (Ontario, for example, has a Blue Book with such listings.) You can find these in public libraries.

Friends.
You may or may not feel comfortable going to a therapist recommended by a friend. Confidentiality would be the main concern, but if you trust your friend and see that he or she has been helped by a particular therapist, you may feel good about going to

this professional. As noted, successful therapy is so personal that most experts in mental health will tell you *not* to use "hairdresser rules" for therapists, but whether to or not often depends on the circumstances. You should be careful about "gurus" or people who seem to have a tremendous influence on the friend who has been helped. There are a variety of cult-like therapists with no formal training who play dangerous mind games with the vulnerable. Look for credentials! This is not to say that only people with credentials are valid therapists, but credentials guarantee that the therapist has had some formal training and is adhering to some code of ethics.

The Phone Book.
You can find plenty of therapists in private practice. These therapists should advertise their credentials up front. If you don't see appropriate degrees after a name, you'd be right to question whether the therapist has any formal training in therapy.

Looking for Credentials

When you're shopping for a therapist, you'll find that one of the most confusing words is "doctor." This is because "doctor" can mean either a medical doctor or a Ph.D., which technically stands for "doctor of philosophy." People obtain Ph.D.'s in a number of academic disciplines, ranging from A (as in anthropology) to Z (as in zoology). Furthermore, a trained medical doctor isn't necessarily a psychiatrist or a trained therapist, either.

An interesting example of credential confusion is the education of Dr. Laura Schlessinger, the host of a popular internationally syndicated radio show. Most people assume that Dr. Laura is either a psychologist or a psychiatrist, but if you look at her credentials, you'll see that she obtained her Ph.D. in physiology, and according to the back cover of one of her books, she also holds "postdoctoral certification and licensing in marriage and family therapy." In other words, Dr. Laura's Ph.D. isn't in the area of mental health. This does not mean that she isn't qualified, however, for after completing her Ph.D., she indeed took the same certification courses that other therapists often take, many of whom don't hold Ph.D.'s. But because "doctor" can be slid in front of her name, the power of the title suggests that she holds more credentials in the field of therapy than she actually does.

Even the "right" letters don't mean that a therapist is properly trained in therapy. For example, a social worker can obtain a master of social work (M.S.W.) degree by taking some general courses in social work theory, but may not have any training specifically related to counselling or therapy. Or, a social worker may have spent most of his or her professional life in work related to policy, having had no exposure to counselling or therapy. Letters may also be meaningless if the therapist obtained them through a disreputable university, college, or society.

But looking at letters is certainly a start. It's a way to help you sort out what sort of training your therapist has likely received. The following professionals should have the corresponding credentials:

Psychiatrist.

A psychiatrist is a medical doctor who specializes in the medical treatment of mental illness and is able to prescribe drugs. Many psychiatrists also do psychotherapy, but this isn't always the case. The appropriate credentials should read: Jane Doe, M.D. (medical doctor), F.R.C.P. (Fellow, Royal College of Physicians). That means this doctor has gone through four years of medical school; has completed a residency program in psychiatry that, depending on the province or territory, lasted approximately four years; and is registered in the Royal College of Physicians and Surgeons.

Psychologist and Psychological Associate.

A psychologist or psychological associate is someone with either a master's degree or doctoral degree who can be licensed to practise therapy. Clinical psychologists have a master of science degree (M.Sc.) or a master of arts (M.A.), and can also hold a Ph.D. (doctor of philosophy) in psychology, an Ed.D. (doctor of education), or, if they're American, a Psy.D. (doctor of psychology), a common degree in the United States. They usually work in a hospital or clinic setting, but can also be found in private practice. Psychologists often perform testing, do assessments, and plan treatments. They can also do psychotherapy, they may have hospital admitting privileges, and they should be registered in the College of Psychologists. In most provinces, someone calling him/herself a "psychologist" would have to be registered or licensed by a provincial body, which isn't necessarily meaningful unless the psychologist worked in a certain kind of setting. The problem with licences is that someone could be well trained as a psychotherapist, with a Ph.D. in psychology, but not be registered with the province, while someone who has no training as a psychotherapist but is, for example, an experimental psychologist (having, say, spent most of his/her professional life with white mice) could call his/herself registered. In some U.S. states, psychologists can also prescribe drugs (a fact you should know in case you need to seek out help while spending time in the U.S.).

Social Worker.

A social worker holds a B.S.W. (bachelor of social work) and/or an M.S.W. (master of social work) and might have completed a bachelor degree in another discipline (which is not at all uncommon). Some social workers have Ph.D.'s as well. The designation "C.S.W." stands for Certified Social Worker, a designation given by the College of Social Work to say that this person is certified and meets the standards required to be a member of the college. In order to obtain a C.S.W., the candidate must write exams and undergo supervision. Social workers can provide counselling and psychotherapy, but it's important to ask your social worker what specific training she or he has had in the area of mental health.

Psychiatric Nurse.

A psychiatric nurse is usually a registered nurse (R.N.) with a bachelor of science in nursing (B.Sc.—a degree that's not absolutely mandatory) who has, but doesn't necessarily require, a master's degree in nursing, too. The master's degree could be either an M.A. or an M.Sc. (master of science). This nurse has done most of his or her training in a psychiatric setting and may be trained to do psychotherapy.

Counsellor.

A counsellor has usually completed certification courses in counselling and therefore has obtained a licence to practise psychotherapy; she or he may have, but does not require, a university degree. Frequently, though, counsellors have a master's degree in a related field, such as social work, or they might have a master's degree in a field unrelated to mental health. The bad news is that there are no official credentials required of a counsellor; that is, there is no legal regulation of the term. Nevertheless, while a television repairperson can, in theory, set up a counselling practice, it's unlikely you'll encounter this. There are various provincial societies and associations to which counsellors may belong, but membership and/or affiliation has little to do with this professional's skill as a therapist. For example, a counsellor living in Toronto may have a business card stating that she is a member of the Ontario Society of Psychotherapy, but that doesn't mean she is a good psychotherapist; it does mean, however, that she is upholding certain standards of practice in order to be a member. It's always a good idea to ask your counsellor what training she or he has had in the field of mental health.

Marriage and Family Counsellor.

"Marriage and family counsellor" has a somewhat different meaning than the broader term "counsellor." This professional has completed rigorous training through certification courses in family therapy and relationship dynamics, and has obtained a licence to practise psychotherapy. He or she may or may not have a master's degree or Ph.D. in a related field, but should have the designations OAFMT (Ontario Association of Family and Marital Therapy) or AAMFT (American Association of Marriage and Family Therapy) after his or her name.

A Word about Fees

It is important to discuss fees with your therapist up front so that you'll know which services are covered by the province or your health plan and which are not. In general, mental health services in hospitals and services provided by psychiatrists are covered by the province. But social workers or counsellors in private practice are all fee-for-service. Call your provincial College of Social Work to determine what a social worker or counsellor in private practice should be charging. If you want to see someone in private practice but can't afford to pay, you might try community-provided counselling services, which are based on your ability to pay. Experts consulted for this book agreed that it is considered bad practice for a counsellor to agree to see someone who cannot (or will not) pay for his or her services. This counsellor is offering a service, not a charity, and the professional relationship should be respected.

Going for a Test Drive

Okay. You found someone you think is qualified to be your therapist. But think again. A qualified therapist isn't necessarily the right therapist for *you*. When you first sit down with this therapist, ask yourself the questions presented below. If you find that you're answering no to many of the questions, you should ask yourself whether you're really with the right therapist. There is no magic number of no's here, but the exercise will help you gauge how you truly feel about the therapist.

1. Do you feel comfortable with this person?

2. Is this someone you can trust?

3. Do you feel calm with this person?

4. Do you feel safe with this person?

5. Does this person respect you (or treat you with respect)?

6. Does this person seem flexible?

7. Does this person seem reliable?

8. Does this person seem supportive?

9. Does this person have a supervisor or mentor with whom they consult on difficult or challenging cases?

Red Flags

You should be cautious about engaging a therapist under any of the following circumstances:

- The therapist does not do a formal assessment, known as a work-up, ruling out organic causes for your symptoms (e.g., thyroid disease). If your therapist is not a physician, she or he may not be trained to do as formal an examination as a physician, but may still be an excellent therapist. However, a therapist *should* ask you where you've been prior to this appointment, and at least inquire about whether you've had a physical examination.

- In the case of a medical doctor or psychiatrist, he or she prescribes antidepressants or other medications upon your first visit. This may be warranted in some circumstances, however. Many psychiatrists will make a decision about medication on a first visit if you've already been seen by another physician or counsellor. But as a general rule, some sort of work-up and discussion is necessary before you are handed a prescription and sent home.

- You are diagnosed or "labelled" with a disorder of some sort within a few minutes of your first visit. Such a situation should only occur if your therapist is a medical doctor. Again, you may be clearly suffering from an identifiable mood disorder, but some discussion and work-up should take place before the diagnosis.

- He or she is adamantly opposed to prescribing any sort of medication, no matter what (this isn't good either; some people require both medication and talk therapy).

- He or she believes in only one approach or theory and seems inflexible with respect to any other approach, theory, or school of thought (a woman-centred approach, for example). This is okay if the therapist is frank about this and clearly explains the advantages and limitations of his or her approach. In this case, you've been informed about the pros and cons and are free to decide if this one-school-of-thought approach is for you.

- She or he does not ask you about your relationships, education, employment, or other aspects of your personal history.

- She or he uses a lot of complicated jargon or technical language that intimidates you. (How can you possibly be expected to talk to someone when you can't understand what she or he is saying?)
- He or she suggests you have sex with him or her to work through your sexual problems. (This is malpractice and should be reported. And yes, women can abuse women, although it is rare.)

Does the Age or Lifestyle of Your Therapist Matter?

The only time the age or lifestyle of your therapist matters is when it matters to *you*, because then it will affect your degree of comfort with that therapist. Although younger therapists certainly have less life experience than older therapists, everyone knows that there are as many wise 31-year-olds as there are 56-year-olds with little wisdom. Younger therapists may be more flexible and caring, less burnt out, and more up-to-date in terms of codes of practice and ethics. Although older therapists may be more rigid in their approach, they have more experience and may be more sensitive to fears of death or aging than younger therapists.

And there are other things to consider. A childless therapist, for example, may be less apt to understand the stresses of a woman with children. Gender preference may also be a factor. If you're a lesbian, you may be more comfortable with a therapist who is gay or lesbian because you want the automatic feeling of acceptance. However, finding someone who is similar to you in some ways isn't a guarantee that you've found the right therapist. Other dynamics are also important: you may be uncomfortable with a father figure or a mother figure; you may be equally uncomfortable with someone the same age as your son or daughter. Although most people strive to find a peer in a therapist, the therapist and the client are not "equal" in this context. In other words, trying to find someone who is much like yourself may not be the best approach when you're looking for a therapist; that's because there is enormous value in there being the right therapeutic distance between you and your therapist.

Styles of Therapy

All of the following styles of therapy can help with stress-related anxiety, panic, or depression. I've listed these not in order of importance, but simply alphabetically.

Biologically Informed Psychotherapy

First, only medical doctors would practise biologically informed psychotherapy because only medical doctors can prescribe medication. This style of therapy is "biopsychiatry," an approach that uses medication in combination with talk therapy. (If you are believed to suffer from seasonal depression, or SAD [seasonal affective disorder], light therapy may be used instead of medication.)

This doesn't mean your therapist is against "talk therapy," however. The therapist who practises biopsychiatry may combine one of the styles of therapy discussed below with medication. But instead of seeing your anxiety or depression stemming solely from a social situation, the therapist will see it as a side-effect of a mood disorder, which is viewed as a medical condition. If you are thinking about suicide, rather than looking at events or situations in your life that might be triggering this thought or desire, a therapist from this school would say, "That's your depression talking [i.e. your disordered brain chemistry], not *you.*" Your anxiety or depression is separated from your circumstances and treated like a medical condition, such as pneumonia. The belief is that once your brain chemistry is "restored," you will begin to think reasonably again and may even be able or willing to shift your perspective on life, which could be done through talk therapy.

This is not unlike an approach used to treat anorexia nervosa. A woman suffering from anorexia might benefit enormously from talk therapy, but if she weighs under 60 pounds and is starving, there is no way for her to "hear" what is being said, let alone participate in talk therapy. She will therefore need to be fed and physically restored before she can hear anything.

If you are incapacitated by your depression, for example, and cannot get out of bed, talk therapy is not useful; the main goal of your therapist at this point would be to "restore" your brain chemistry and *get you out of bed.* This may be done through antidepressant medication, for example. In biopsychiatry, the therapist doesn't believe that medication can fix everything; rather that it can facilitate productive talk therapy.

Cognitive-Behavioural Therapy

Cognitive-behavioural therapy is oriented toward upbeat thinking and correcting what is referred to as "disordered thinking." It doesn't focus on the client's negative thoughts but instead is based on the premise "How you think can affect how you feel." For example, if a friend cancels a lunch date with you, you may take it personally and assume that your friend is angry with you. That thought then leads you to feel badly about yourself, reinforcing feelings of low self-esteem or even self-loathing. A cognitive-behavioural therapist will ask you to consider other reasons for the cancellation. Perhaps your friend is overwhelmed by problems and stresses that have absolutely nothing to do with you. Perhaps a last-minute deadline came up that necessitated the cancellation. In other words, not everything you perceive to be negative is really negative, and not everything you take personally is personal.

Ultimately, the premise of cognitive-behavioural therapy is this: if you think negative thoughts about yourself and believe that you're a failure or that your life is doomed, you are more apt to be anxious, depressed, or sad. On the other hand, if you think positive thoughts and believe in yourself, you are more apt to be happy. Although this might sound like an easy, quick-fix approach, changing your perspective on life can be a powerful remedy. But again, in the midst of a depression, this sort of effort may have limited success. It's important to remember, however, that what's past is past; you can decide *today* to be a more positive person, and a more positive attitude, in turn, can bring more positive experiences into your life.

Cognitive therapy is especially beneficial for people suffering from panic attacks, as I discussed earlier. This style of therapy can teach you to anticipate the situations and bodily sensations that are associated with panic attacks; having this awareness can actually help you to control the attacks. You can also do any one of a number of mental exercises to keep from hyperventilating or having fearful thoughts. For instance, by replacing the thought "I'm dying" with "I'm just hyperventilating—I can handle this," you'll be able to calm the panic attack before the unchecked fear takes over and the symptoms worsen.

Feminist Therapy

Feminist therapy is woman-centred therapy. When looking at the symptoms that comprise women's stress—anxiety, panic, and depression—the feminist therapist does not apply just one specific style of therapy, but an overall philosophy of therapy that takes women's social roles and social situations into account. In a nutshell, a feminist therapist appreciates that you can't win a dog show when you're a cat! Careful: I am not saying that this is the only suitable style of therapy for women. And plenty of female therapists do *not* embrace feminist therapy. In general, the feminist therapist hopes that the women she treats will achieve the following goals:

1. Develop a sense of self, independent of male authority or idealized visions of what a woman is supposed to be. A woman's task is not to develop a male

persona but to celebrate her own feminine persona and see her traits as important human virtues rather than as liabilities in a male world.

2. Understand that "the personal is political," as the adage goes. Feminist therapists listen for the connections between the personal story and the outer world in women's lives. The therapist uses feminist values to help shift a woman from seeing herself as a victim to seeing how the world *around* her is creating her feelings of victimization—a change of perception that is validating.

3. See that depression is really the internalization of oppression. (This does not mean, however, that you should just walk around depressed and not seek out help.)

4. See that feelings of low self-esteem, worthlessness, inadequacy, powerlessness, poor body image, anxiety, depression, and/or sexual dysfunction are symptoms of female subservience in a man's world. In other words, they are normal, adaptive responses to the world around you, rather than symptoms of a disease or sickness. (Again, this does not mean that you should accept as inevitable your feelings of depression, low self-esteem, and so on, and not get help. In other words, cold symptoms may be normal reactions to a common cold virus, but you still need to care for yourself by resting and drinking plenty of fluids to get better.)

5. Understand that self-sacrificing behaviour is normal feminine, nurturing behaviour, not a symptom of disease. Labels such as "co-dependent" are not helpful and should be dismissed as psychobabble.

6. See that physical ailments are valid and should be trusted as another way of "knowing." In other words, women's bodies may be trying to tell them something about the environment or the toxic lifestyle to which they have become numb. For example, many women who have chronic fatigue or environmental sensitivities should see their symptoms as visionary or intuitive, rather than as invalid or phantom. As discussed at the beginning of this chapter, there is a link between feminine intuition, ecology, and environment, one that's recognized in the ecofeminism field of study. Women's physical ailment and body intuition have too often been dismissed, to the world's peril.

7. See that human emotional pain is not a medical problem but a normal response to one's environment. In other words, pain in response to a bad situation is normal, not sick.

8. Understand that grief is grief. Grieving over the death of a loved one is not different from grieving over one's poverty or life circumstances. Yet, in the medical

world, some things are more worthy of grief than others, which means that you are labelled "normal" for some kinds of grieving but "sick" for others.

9. See yourself as connected to all women. What you suffer, other women suffer. You are not alone, but part of a community. The solution cannot be found on an individual level but must be arrived at collectively. For example, one black person in 1950 could not overturn centuries of racism and segregation. It took a movement, not a single individual.

A therapist doesn't have to be female to offer a woman-centred approach. If you are interested in seeking the help of a feminist therapist, the best places to contact for names are women's centres; you might even try women's studies programs at local universities.

Interpersonal Therapy

Interpersonal therapy is a very specific approach to therapy based on the idea that malfunctioning relationships are behind your symptoms of anxiety or depression. In other words, where there's anxiety and depression, there are also dysfunctional relationships that interfere with the quality of life. You and your therapist will explore current relationships and recent events that may have affected those relationships, such as loss, conflict, or change. You may also explore the roles that various people are playing in your life, what your expectations are of these people, and vice versa. Your therapist works in a supporting role, helping you to resolve conflicts by developing better strategies to cope or negotiate with the key people in your life. Much of this has to do with setting reasonable expectations for your relationships and looking at how you might have misinterpreted the actions of others.

Psychoanalysis

It's important not to confuse psychoanalysis with psychoanalytic therapy. The latter is more along the lines of psychodynamic therapy (see below), while psychoanalysis is an intensive therapy that usually involves daily sessions and is not recommended for people with depression who are unable to function well. This therapy works best when the crisis has passed, and thus suits people who are ready for self-discovery. Based on the premise that the problems you have today stem from wounds you suffered as a child, it is a journey into your childhood. For example, you may be seeking to gratify in your adult life the unmet needs you had as a child. Or you may discover that behaviour from your childhood, such as "pleasing your parents," is being re-enacted in your workplace or in your personal relationships. Women who underwent psychoanalysis in the past were frequently harmed because the therapy tended to reinforce father-figure/little-girl relationships. Today, if properly done, psychoanalysis is not something women have to fear, and many excellent psychoanalysts are women.

Psychodynamic Therapy

Psychodynamic therapy deals with "ghosts," relationships, and events from your past, the dynamics of your upbringing, as well as present events and relationships. Here, your thoughts, emotions, and behaviour over a lifetime are examined, and patterns of behaviour and aspects of your personality are discussed as possible sources of both internal and external conflict. Couples or groups are often involved in psychodynamic therapy. The adage "The past is history, the future a mystery, and the present a gift" works well in this context.

3
STRESS AGGRAVATORS

When women are under stress, they often self-medicate with cigarettes, alcohol, prescription drugs, or illegal substances. Other things in our diet—such as caffeine— or just our dieting behaviour (binging, purging, or starving) can badly aggravate stress. This chapter walks you through all of the stress aggravators. Self-medicating both the physical and emotional signs of stress begins by removing the "self-medications" that are making you feel worse.

Women and Cigarettes

Many women turn to cigarettes to deal with the demands of stress, but studies show that people who smoke every day are twice as likely to suffer from depression—which can be triggered by stress—as people who don't smoke. The depression may have nothing to do with smoking and *everything* to do with stressful circumstances. In other words, people under a lot of stress are more likely to suffer from depression, and a great many of those people are likely to smoke to try to calm themselves. Other studies have found that people with major depression are three times as likely to be daily smokers as people without major depression. It's possible that nicotine is a drug we crave in order to medicate our depressed moods.

Smoking also satisfies "mouth hunger"—the need to have something in your mouth—which often occurs during stressful periods. Women who are afraid that their stress will drive them to food often turn to cigarettes instead. Stress can also turn a social smoker into a much heavier smoker or even into a chain smoker. It becomes a bit of a no-win cycle when women try to cut down, because the withdrawal symptoms can drive women to food as well, which only makes them smoke more.

In the 1920s, medical journals and the medical profession recommended smoking to women as a way to "calm" themselves. The idea of controlling weight with cigarettes also emerged at that time. When a tobacco company wife was told by her doctor to smoke to "relax," she found that smoking not only relaxed her, but actually helped to curb her appetite. Thus began the luring of women to cigarettes.

> I started smoking when I was 15 because I felt fat and ugly compared to all my girlfriends. I wanted to look like Madonna, who was very popular at that time. I thought I would lose weight if I smoked. I would smoke only outside the house, so my parents never knew. When I got into university, I started to see this wonderful guy who wanted me to quit; he complained of the way I tasted and smelled. I didn't think that quitting would be so difficult, but I just couldn't withstand the cravings. I never quit, and I tried to mask my smoking with gum or mouthwash. It didn't fool him and he said that he just couldn't date a smoker. I was very sad that I couldn't come through for him, and I still think about him. My smoking has increased over the years, and I find that the older I get and the more stress I take on at work, the more I want to smoke. In a strange way, it feels like the only guaranteed pleasure in life, since I feel so much of my life is just boring and nothing special—I'm single, still overweight, and hate my job. I look forward to smoking; it helps me get through the day.

You've no doubt been bombarded with information about the health consequences of smoking, but many of you probably don't realize this alarming, yet under-reported fact: *the number one killer of women is cigarettes and smoking.* Smoking-related diseases directly kill more women than any other health or social problem. Worse, people who don't smoke get sick from environmental tobacco smoke. And yet smoking remains legal. The number one killer of women is smoking-related lung cancer; next come smoking-related heart disease, smoking-related stroke, and smoking-related chronic lung diseases (very common yet under-reported). And did you know that early menopause and osteoporosis are more common among smokers? Then there are the top killer cancers in the general population that are more prevalent in women who smoke—colon cancer and breast cancer—as well as a range of gynecological and gastrointestinal cancers now on the rise. And what's more, even though the rates of cervical cancer have dropped, smokers are more susceptible to this cancer than non-smokers. *If you smoke and are under stress, you have an even greater chance of developing one or some of the above.*

All studies show that women who smoke "get sicker quicker." They develop, and die from, smoking-related diseases at much younger ages than men. It's not unusual for women in their 30s to develop lung cancer, for example. If you compare a man and a woman with similar smoking habits, the woman is twice as likely to die. Yet women are smoking in increasing numbers. More shocking, 20 to 25 percent of pregnant women continue to smoke during their pregnancies.

A single cigarette affects your body within seconds, increasing your heart rate, blood pressure, and the demand for oxygen. The greater the demand for oxygen (because of constricted blood vessels and carbon monoxide, a by-product of cigarettes), the greater the risk of heart disease. Lesser-known long-term effects of smoking include a lowering of HDL, or "good" cholesterol, and damage to the lining of blood vessel walls, paving the way for a host of stress-related illnesses.

Marketing "Violence" against Women

I'm not giving you all this bad news because I want you to feel worse; I'm telling you this to make you aware of a dangerous predator: tobacco companies. Make no mistake—the tobacco companies specifically target women. Right now, this predator is out to kill you and your daughters, nieces, and granddaughters. So long as tobacco companies advertise in women's magazines and continue to sponsor sports events and fashion shows, they will remain killers of women.

It's important that women realize that tobacco companies take advantage of young women's body-image dilemmas to addict them early to nicotine; early addiction has devastating health consequences for you the smoker and for your daughter, who may well be smoking when you're not looking. The results of numerous studies show that most young women begin smoking to *control their weight* (see Chapter 6).

Tobacco ads in women's magazines continue to sell the message to young women that smoking is "beautiful" or "glamorous." One brand, as of 1999, sported the copy "It's a woman's thing," showing a beautiful, thin woman in a natural setting.

As the women's movement (also known as second-wave feminism) grew in the 1960s, smoking began to be associated with "independence." By the late 1960s, one in three women in North America smoked. The popular campaign slogan used by Virginia Slims, "You've Come a Long Way, Baby," played up this independence theme, a theme that seemed to attract women to cigarettes like moths to a flame.

Tobacco companies continue to target women in their advertisements, aiming especially at international markets, where rates of women smokers are much lower.

They use Western "glamour" in their ads to entice women in developing countries to smoke—women whose health risks are greater due to extreme poverty and poor access to health care.

In effect, these tobacco ads are marketing a form of violence against women. It's no better on a moral scale than a man luring a woman into his apartment and then raping and killing her.

It's Enough to Make You Quit

Don't let the tobacco companies win! Get mad and take back your life. When smokers hear the following facts, many of them get so angry, they quit. So I tell you these things not to punish you, but to motivate you. It's been long known that unethical practices such as the following go on in the tobacco industry:

- The suppression of evidence linking tobacco with ill health.
- The use of nicotine to enhance the addictive properties of tobacco. Cigarette manufacturing, in this case, becomes all about "nicotine delivery."
- The circulation of misleading information that masks the health consequences of smoking.
- The use of advertising that targets vulnerable groups. These ad campaigns sink to terrible lows in their intent to appeal to children, young women, and low-income individuals.
- The export of tobacco products to Third World nations, often with accompanying advertising aimed at minors or other groups who don't have the income to support a nicotine addiction.

Take a look at some of the things you'll gain by quitting smoking:

- Decreased risk of heart disease
- Decreased risk of cancer (that includes cancer of the lung, esophagus, mouth, throat, pancreas, kidney, bladder, and cervix)
- Lower heart rate and blood pressure
- Decreased risk of lung disease (bronchitis, emphysema)
- Relaxation of blood vessels
- Improved sense of smell and taste
- Better teeth
- Fewer wrinkles

How Women Become Addicted

Without the awareness and decision-making powers of an informed adult, young women are vulnerable targets. Once a young girl buys into the marketing messages delivered to her by tobacco companies (e.g., smoking is glamorous, keeps you thin, etc.) and begins smoking, she's hooked. Here's why.

Nicotine produces a "controlled" response, and thus the smoker can either stimulate herself or calm herself. Small, shallow puffs on a cigarette enable a smoker to keep awake, alert, or active when she is fatigued, allowing her to more easily shoulder her "double duties." Deep drags from a cigarette give the smoker larger doses of nicotine, facilitating the release of endorphins, "feel good" chemicals that the body makes. Endorphins are naturally released when we laugh, exercise, and do anything pleasurable, like eating something tasty. Since the endorphins come from the body naturally, smokers find that they do, in fact, perform better and are less stressed when they smoke more. On drugs such as amphetamines, heroine, or cocaine, the high is produced by the drug, not the body, so it feels completely different. Nicotine does not feel like a drug in the same way.

What is addictive is the control the cigarette gives a woman: shallow puffs = stimulant; deep drags = relaxation. All studies on women smokers reveal that the more stress a woman is under, the more she will smoke. Smoking can allow a woman to endure much more stress, and that adds up to a real physical toll on the body. We already know that stress is hard on the body; more smoking is also hard on the body, producing a "double whammy" physically.

Why Quitting Is So Hard

Within 7 to 10 seconds after you've inhaled cigarette, a concentrated dose of nicotine goes directly to your brain, producing a "rush" that, in turn, stimulates the release of a number of neurotransmitters (or "messengers"), including dopamine and noradrenaline, a stress hormone.

When a woman tries to quit smoking, dopamine and noradrenaline levels drop, and that produces a strong urge to smoke in addition to withdrawal symptoms such as anxiety, depression, irritability, insomnia, difficulty concentrating, increased appetite, gastrointestinal discomfort, headaches, and lightheadedness. These withdrawal symptoms can actually worsen over a week, rather than lessen. The cravings can last for months. Most women begin to smoke again to relieve the suffering—especially during periods of high stress.

Why Girls Start Smoking

Studies show that eating disorders and smoking are intricately linked. Young girls reveal that when they are feeling "fat" or "ugly," they will smoke to cope with these negative feelings; they will smoke, too, to cut down on their eating.

Young girls also turn to smoking when, through various social experiences with sexism or unfair situations that appear to favour men, they begin to figure out that the world was not built for women. This realization leads them into a kind of social withdrawal; smoking helps them cope with the social awkwardness they feel from just being female in this culture.

What about "Light" Cigarettes?

In the 1960s, when health warnings about smoking were beginning to be issued, the tobacco industry introduced "light" or "low tar" cigarettes. These were meant to appeal to women specifically, and women did buy them in record numbers. Both those who wanted to quit smoking and those who wanted to avoid the health risks of smoking bought into the lie that a "lighter" cigarette is less harmful and therefore "healthier." *This is completely false.* All cigarettes are made to deliver enough nicotine to keep you addicted. A light cigarette may be altered in that it has a different smell or appears less dense, but all of the research on light cigarettes since the 1980s has found that when smokers switch to a light cigarette, they get the same dose of nicotine because they take deeper drags and actually hold the smoke in their lungs longer. In short, women who smoke light cigarettes wind up smoking more rather than less. More recent research has linked some forms of cancer to the smoking of light cigarettes.

Take a Look at What You're Inhaling

In 1989 the U.S. surgeon general released a report listing 43 carcinogenic agents found in tobacco smoke. The IARC (International Agency for Research on Cancer) classified them as follows.

TABLE 3.1   Carcinogenic Agents Found in Tobacco Smoke

Group 1A: Carcinogenic to Humans

Tobacco smoke	2-Naphthylamine
Tobacco products, smokeless	Nickel
4-Aminobuphenyl	Polonium
Benzene	Nickel
Cadmium	Polonium-210 (radon)
Chromium	Vinyl chloride

Group 2A: Probably Carcinogenic to Humans

Acrylonitrile	Dibenz[a,h]anthracene
Benzo[a]anthracene	Formaldehyde
Benzo[a]pyrene	N-Nitrosodiethylamine
1,3-Butadine	N-Nitrosodimethlamine

Group 2B: Possibly Carcinogenic to Humans

Acetaldehyde	Lead
Benzo[b]fluoranthene	5-Methylchrysene
Benzo[j]fluoranthene	4-(Methylnitrosamine)-2-(3-pyridyl)-1-butanene (NNK)
Benzo[k]fluoranthene	
Dibenz[a,h]acridine	2-Nitropropane
Dibenz[a,j]acridine	N-Nitrosodiethanolamine
7H-Dibenz[c,g]carbazole	N-Nitrosomethylethylamine
Dibenzo[a,l]pyrene	N-Nitrosomorpholine
1,1-Dimethylhydrazine	N-Nitrosopyrrolidine
Hydrazine	Quinoline
Indeno-2,3[c,d]pyrene	Ortho-toluidine
	Urethane (ethyl carbamate)

Group 3: Unclassified as to Carcinogenicity to Humans (Limited Evidence)

Chrysene	N-Nitrosoanabasine (NAB)
Crotonaldehyde	N-Nitrosoanatabine (NAT)

Quitting Stress-Related Smoking

Therapists specializing in smoking-cessation programs for women report that women refer to cigarettes as their "best friend" and say that they mourn the loss of this friend when they try to quit. Women also see a cigarette as their "reward." The smoking break is seen as "earned" by hard work or stress. Replacing the reward with something else that meets a woman's psychological and spiritual needs is imperative if she is to succeed in quitting. The success rate for quitting triples for women who have sought out specific smoking-cessation counselling.

Herbal and Homeopathic Smoking-Cessation Aids.

There are many herbal and homeopathic smoking-cessation products. Some use plant sources to reduce cravings; some work by using natural substances to help you "detox." For information on the many natural smoking-cessation products available in Canada, contact Canada's leading natural pharmacy, Smith's Pharmacy, at 1-800-361-6624, or visit the pharmacy's website, **www.smithspharmacy.com**.

Behavioural Counselling.

Behavioural counselling, either group or individual, can raise the rate of abstinence to 20–25 percent. This approach to smoking cessation aims to change the mental processes of the smoker, reinforce the benefits of non-smoking, and teach the smoker how to avoid the urge to smoke.

Nicotine Gum.

Nicotine (Nicorette) gum is now available over the counter. It helps you quit smoking by reducing the nicotine cravings and withdrawal symptoms once you've stopped smoking. Nicotine gum helps you wean yourself from nicotine by allowing you to gradually decrease the dosage until you stop using it altogether, a process that usually takes about 12 weeks. The only disadvantage with this method is that it caters to the oral and addictive aspects of smoking (i.e., rewarding the urge to smoke with a dose of nicotine).

Nicotine Patch.

Transdermal nicotine, or the "patch" (Habitrol, Nicoderm, Nicotrol), doubles abstinence rates in former smokers. Most brands are now available over the counter. Each morning, you apply a new patch to a different area of dry, clean, hairless skin and leave it on for the day. Some patches are designed to be worn a full 24 hours. However, the constant supply of nicotine to the bloodstream sometimes causes very vivid or disturbing dreams. You can also expect to feel a mild itching, burning, or tingling at the site of the patch when it is first applied. The nicotine patch works best when it is worn for at least 7 to 12 weeks, with a gradual decrease in strength (i.e., nicotine). Many smokers find it effective because it allows them to tackle their psychological addiction to smoking before they are forced to deal with the physical symptoms of withdrawal.

Nicotine Inhaler.

The nicotine inhaler (Nicotrol Inhaler) delivers nicotine orally via inhalation from a plastic tube. Its success rate is about 28 percent, similar to that of nicotine gum. As of this writing, it's available by prescription only in the United States and has yet to make its debut in Canada. Like nicotine gum, the inhaler mimics smoking behaviour because you can respond to each craving or urge to smoke by taking a "puff," a feature that has both advantages and disadvantages to the smoker who wants to get over the physical symptoms of withdrawal. The nicotine inhaler should be used for a period of 12 weeks.

Nicotine Nasal Spray.

Like nicotine gum and the nicotine patch, the nasal spray reduces craving and withdrawal symptoms, allowing smokers to cut back gradually. One squirt delivers about 1 mg of nicotine. In three clinical trials involving 730 patients, 31–35 percent were not smoking at six months. This compares to an average of 12–15 percent of smokers who were able to quit unaided. The nasal spray has a couple of advantages over the gum and the patch: nicotine is rapidly absorbed across the nasal membranes, providing a kick that is more like the real thing, and the prompt onset of action, plus a flexible dosing schedule, benefits heavier smokers. Because the nicotine reaches your bloodstream so quickly, nasal sprays do have a greater potential for addiction than the slower-acting gum and patch. As of this writing, nasal sprays are not yet available for use in Canada.

Alternative Therapies.

Hypnosis, meditation, and acupuncture have helped some smokers quit. In the case of hypnosis and meditation, sessions may be private or part of a group smoking-cessation program.

Smoking-Cessation Drugs

The drug bupropion (Zyban) is now available and is an option for people who have been unsuccessful using nicotine replacement. Formerly prescribed as an antidepressant, bupropion was discovered by accident: researchers knew that smokers trying to quit were often depressed, so they began experimenting with the drug as a means to fight depression, not addiction. Bupropion reduces the withdrawal symptoms associated with smoking cessation and can be used in conjunction with nicotine-replacement therapy. Researchers suspect that the drug works directly in the brain, disrupting the addictive power of nicotine by affecting the same chemical neuro-transmitters in the brain that nicotine does (e.g., dopamine).

The pleasurable aspect of addictive drugs like nicotine and cocaine is triggered by the release of dopamine. Smoking floods the brain with dopamine. The *New England Journal of Medicine* published the results of a study involving more than 600 smokers taking bupropion. At the end of treatment, 44 percent of those who took the highest dose of the drug (300 mg) were not smoking, compared to a 19 percent success rate for those of the group who took a placebo. By the end of one year, 23 percent of the 300 mg group and 12 percent of the placebo group were still not smoking. Using Zyban *with* nicotine-replacement therapy seems to improve the quit rate a bit further. Four-week quit rates from the study were 23 percent for placebo, 36 percent for the patch, 49 percent for Zyban, and 58 percent for the combination of Zyban and the patch.

Women and Cigars

Cigar smoking is in vogue for women who want to be perceived as in the "know," in the "money," or "cool." And it is a dangerous trend that is capturing the interest of millions of women in higher income brackets. When you smoke a cigar, you're getting filler, binder, and wrapper, all of which are made of air-cured and fermented tobac-cos. Like cigarette tobacco, lit cigars emit over 4,000 chemicals, 43 of which are known to cause cancer.

Cigar smokers have higher death rates than non-smokers for most smoking-related diseases, although rates for cigar smokers are not nearly as high as for cigar-ette smokers. Because the nicotine is absorbed through the mouth, however, cigar/pipe smokers, as well as anyone using chewing tobacco or snuff, are at higher risk for laryngeal, oral, and esophageal cancer. Cigar/pipe smokers also have higher death rates than non-smokers from chronic obstructive lung disease as well as lung cancer.

Women are being sold cigar smoking as a pastime that is attractive and sexy. And women are actually buying into it when they are, in fact, perhaps unconsciously, much more attracted to the maleness of the cigar and the "male world" it seems to evoke for them. As one health promotion expert relayed to me, "A cigar is *not* just a cigar—it's the same death trap with a bigger penis."

Wine, Women, and Drinking Problems

I need my wine every night. Not a whole bottle—just two or three glasses a night. If you want to label me an alcoholic then I would counter with the term "highly functional alcoholic." It doesn't interfere with my life, it's just something I really enjoy, look forward to, and need to have waiting when I come home. My boyfriend doesn't join me when I drink; he judges me, and he will often voice his disapproval. One day I said to him, "You know what …? I'll replace you before I replace my wine!"

Surveys reveal that by 2004, North American women will consume an average of eight drinks per week. Many women first develop a drinking problem (which is different than drinking wine when out for dinner or socializing) during a crisis or while under stress. Women who self-medicate with alcohol can develop health problems with lower levels of drinking over a shorter period of time than men who self-medicate in this way. Women also tend to be silent drinkers, drinking alone. Moderate drinking is defined as being less than 12 drinks per week and not on a daily basis. Moderate drinkers do not use alcohol to cope with stress, nor do they plan their recreational activities around alcohol. If you think you're drinking more heavily, keeping a diary of your drinking is useful. Just being aware of your alcohol consumption patterns can be enough for you to change your habits.

Two key facts emerge from all of the academic articles on women and alcohol abuse: women drink for completely different reasons than men, and the Alcoholics Anonymous 12-step programs are usually not successful ways for women to stop drinking (these programs were modelled after male patterns of alcoholism). Women who drink come from a range of educational and economic backgrounds. A highly educated woman is just as likely to begin drinking as a woman with no education; in fact, the more education a woman has, the more *likely* she is to begin drinking as she ages.

Women often use alcohol to improve their sexual relationships; they typically use alcohol to overcome their inhibitions so that they can fully express their passions and feelings. Men, however, tend to use alcohol to numb their feelings. Many women cannot function sexually without drinking first to loosen up. They use the bottle to come *out* of the bottle. Women are more likely to drink wine rather than hard liquor, while men tend to use "the hard stuff" to get drunk fast.

For the most part, you'll read different statistics about the woman alcoholic. She may be portrayed as having a dependent personality, as being more likely to suffer from depression, or as coming from a family of alcoholics. But for the most accurate take on women and alcohol, go to your local video store. Most of what you need to know about women and drinking you'll find already captured on film in movies such as *The Days of Wine and Roses* (originally a teleplay starring Cliff Robertson and Piper Laurie, but in 1960 made into a film starring Jack Lemmon and Lee Remick). The woman in *Days* is very passive and sweet; she tells her alcoholic boyfriend that she prefers chocolate to alcohol. So he introduces her into his world through crème de cacao. She likes it very much; she finds a new voice through the alcohol. She becomes witty and sexual. And so it goes until their lives begin to crumble because of their addiction. True to life, he finds salvation through Alcoholics Anonymous; she, on the other hand, doesn't benefit from AA in the way he does. In the end, he is saved and must accept that only she can save herself if she chooses.

For another true-to-life portrayal, slip *Who's Afraid of Virginia Woolf?* into your VCR and watch Elizabeth Taylor and Richard Burton imitate their lives through their art in the film version of Edward Albee's famous play. Both Martha and George are alcoholics. But George uses alcohol to numb his voice and feelings, to forget the past; Martha, on the other hand, uses alcohol to enable herself to voice her frustrations with the past. In front of guests, she blurts out one terrible truth after another about George, their life, and, ultimately, all of her lost dreams. We learn, for example, that she is the daughter of a famous professor and is actually brighter than George; had she been given an opportunity, she could have become as accomplished as her father. Instead, she married George, a mediocre academic who secured a position with the university through Martha's father. An old story. And so true.

Why Women Start Drinking

Women drink to "enable" their voice in a world where they often feel they have no voice. They feel looser and more at ease when drinking. While under stress, many women feel like exploding but restrain themselves; alcohol gives them permission to express all of their anger, their "beefs," and so on. And so the drinking pattern starts. Usually alcohol feels good as an enabler, but because it is, in fact, addictive, it turns into an addiction. Creative women will often use alcohol as a creative enabler, which is why so many women artists have struggled with alcoholism. Alcoholism and depression often go hand in hand, but it is more accurate to say that the depression comes first and the alcohol provides a temporary reprieve from the depression. As I said above, many women drink silently, out of public view; this enables freer thinking, relaxation, and a time for them to let down their guard.

When women become addicted to alcohol, they may become what's known as "cross-addicted"; that is, they combine alcohol with other substances, such as various prescription or illegal drugs. When women become dependent on alcohol, they have an alcohol problem; many women are unaware of their dependence on alcohol, however, because, to them, their alcohol intake appears manageable.

> I started to drink wine in the evenings as a way to unwind. I was thinking: women are just handed prescriptions for antidepressants willy-nilly by doctors and no one questions it—yet all this fuss about drinking alone is made. I mixed up the weekends that my daughter would be staying with me. I got home at around 4:30 one Friday (I left the office early that day in anticipation of my alone time), thinking my ex-husband was picking her up at school. I poured a glass of Chardonnay and went outside on my deck to start relaxing. At 6:00 p.m. the phone rang. It was my daughter calling from school—where was I? "Didn't Dad come?" I asked. When I realized my mistake, I knew there was an even bigger problem—I couldn't drive. I had had two glasses of wine and was already buzzed and sort of tipsy. I called a taxi for my daughter and tried to stuff as many carbs as I could down my throat to absorb the alcohol. I'm not sure that two glasses of wine is that big a problem … but that day, it was a problem for me.

Health Risks of Alcohol

If you tend to use wine or other alcoholic beverages to unwind after a stressful day, be aware that alcohol can interfere with sleep patterns and is also a depressant. Initially, alcohol may make you tired and you therefore may think it's a sleeping aid, but it can wake you up later on, causing you to be wide awake at 2:00 a.m. and preventing you from falling back to sleep. Naturally, all of this can aggravate stress and fatigue.

Women also metabolize alcohol differently than men, so even when a man and woman are the same weight, the woman will become intoxicated more easily than the man—it has to do with fat distribution.

Unlike smoking, alcohol is not directly linked to diseases that specifically kill women. Over the years, studies have shown that women who drink more tend to be more susceptible to breast cancer, although this may have more to do with the calories in alcohol (the link between breast cancer and fat) than with the alcohol itself.

The more immediate health risks of alcohol abuse for women involve liver problems, such as cirrhosis of the liver, and the hangovers caused by overindulgence (hangovers can have a significant impact on overall health and stress). But when women try to seek help, they are often blocked by family members (especially spouses) who would rather leave the problem unacknowledged; there is still a stigma associated with women and alcohol, unlike for women who smoke.

Alcohol and PMS

Alcohol is tolerated by the same woman differently at different times in her cycle. She may become more easily intoxicated just before ovulation, and alcohol can aggravate premenstrual discomforts. Several studies have confirmed that the amount of alcohol you consume directly affects the severity of your premenstrual discomforts. For example, in most (but not all) of the studies that have looked into this link, the women who reported severe PMS were typically found to be the heavier drinkers. However, the more stress in your life, the more likely you are to drink, too, which loops back to the stress-PMS theory discussed in Chapter 1.

Alcohol and Weight Gain

Alcohol delivers about 7 calories per gram or 150 calories per drink. A glass of dry wine with your meal adds about 100 calories. A drink that's half soda water and half wine (a spritzer) contains half the calories. When you cook with wine, the alcohol evaporates, leaving only the flavour. If you're a beer drinker, you're adding about 150 calories per bottle to your meal. A light beer, though "lighter," contains at least 100 calories per bottle.

The stiffer the drink, the fatter it gets. Hard liquor such as scotch, rye, gin, and rum are made out of cereal grains; vodka, the Russian staple, is made out of potatoes. Hard liquor averages about 40 percent alcohol but has no sugar. Nevertheless, you're looking at about 100 calories per small shot glass, so long as you don't add fruit, tomato, or clamato juice or sugary soft drinks.

Dietary Factors

I am considered a fit, healthy person by my friends. But the truth is, when I'm under a lot of stress, I make frequent trips to the McDonald's drive-thru. There's one near my office, and there's one near my home. One day, I found myself there for breakfast, lunch, and dinner—and felt like I had graduated to utter "Loserdom." I'd rather be caught shoplifting than be seen at McDonald's! It's not like I'm getting any of their healthy meals, either! I go right for the "fix"—Egg McMuffins, Quarter Pounders (with cheese), and the staples of my high-stress diet: McDonald's french fries. At times I feel like it's an addiction. I never actually go inside. I always use the drive-thru; I need the anonymity of the car.

Stress can cause us to miss meals or eat on the run, which means we're often eating high-starch foods with very few nutrients. This can aggravate stress because it can make it more difficult for our bodies to maintain stable blood sugar levels—something that directly affects our moods.

Many women suffer from repeated episodes of low blood sugar, a condition known as hypoglycemia. The consumption of too many carbohydrates produces an initial rush of energy that's followed by a tremendous crash, which is sometimes known as post-prandial depression (or post-meal depression). In fact, it's not at all unusual for people who are depressed or under stress to crave starches and sweets, or what's known as simple carbohydrates (complex carbs are grains, fruit, etc.). The problem with simple carbs is that they break down into glucose more quickly; the faster the breakdown into glucose, the faster the drop in blood sugar, leading to a drop in mood. By increasing your intake of protein and fibre, you can help to delay the breakdown of your food into glucose and thus keep your blood sugar levels more stable throughout the day. A nutritionist or dietician can help you select better foods for high-stress times.

Caffeine

Lots of studies show that caffeine causes anxiety and sleeplessness, and is mildly addictive. It also worsens premenstrual discomforts. Health Canada now recommends that you consume no more than 400–450 mg of caffeine per day, which is equal to two 8 oz mugs of gourmet coffee or four cups of instant coffee. Of course, there are many other sources of caffeine—soft drinks, chocolate, tea, and so forth. All sources of caffeine should be taken into account as you follow Health Canada's recommendations.

You should also be aware that caffeine is one of the worst aggravators of stress around. It raises your blood pressure and increases the secretion of adrenaline, one of the stress hormones. Here's a checklist that details how much caffeine some foods/drinks contain, with the milligrams of caffeine in parentheses.

Coffee (5 oz/142 g cup)

Brewed, drip method (60–180 mg)

Brewed, percolator (40–170 mg)

Instant (30–120 mg)

Decaffeinated, brewed (2–5 mg)

Decaffeinated, instant (1–5 mg)

Tea (5 oz/142 g cup)

Brewed, major brands (20–90 mg)

Brewed, imported brands (25–110 mg)

Instant (25–50 mg)

Iced, 12 oz/340 g (67–76 mg)

Other

6 oz/170 g glass of caffeine-containing soft drink (15–30 mg)

5 oz/142 g cup of cocoa beverage (2–20 mg)

8 oz/227 g glass of chocolate milk (2–7 mg)

1 oz/28 g serving of milk chocolate (1–15 mg)

1 oz/28 g serving of dark chocolate, semi-sweet (5–35 mg)

Single square of Baker's chocolate (26 mg)

Serving of chocolate-flavoured syrup (4 mg)

Binge Eating

Stress can induce binge eating, also known as compulsive eating. Many women will turn to food as a comfort during times of stress or when other things are missing in their lives, such as sexual satisfaction, love, or other sensuous aspects of life.

The following is a typical profile of a compulsive eater:

• Eats when she's not hungry

• Feels out of control when she's around food, either trying to resist it or gorging on it

• Spends a lot of time thinking/worrying about food and her weight

• Always desperate to try another diet that promises results

- Has feelings of self-loathing and shame
- Hates her own body
- Obsessed with what she can or will eat, or has eaten
- Eats in secret or with "eating friends"
- Appears to be a professional dieter who's in control
- Buys cakes or pies as "gifts" and has them wrapped to hide the fact that they're for herself
- Has a pristine kitchen with only the "right" foods
- Feels either out of control with food (compulsive eating) or imprisoned by it (dieting)
- Feels temporary relief by "not eating"
- Looks forward with pleasure and anticipation to the time when she can eat alone
- Feels unhappy because of her eating behaviour

Most people eat when they're hungry. For the compulsive eater, hunger cues have nothing to do with when she eats. She may eat for any of the following reasons:

- To satisfy mouth hunger—the need to have something in her mouth, even though she's not hungry
- To prevent *future* hunger: "Better eat now because later I may not get a chance."
- To make up for a bad day or bad experience, or to reward herself for a good day or good experience
- Because "It's the only pleasure I can count on!"
- To quell nerves
- To relieve boredom
- Because she's "going on a diet" tomorrow (hence, the eating is done out of a real fear that she will be deprived later)
- Because food is her friend

Food addiction, like other addictions, can be treated successfully with a 12-step program. The original 12-step program was started in the 1930s by an alcoholic who was able to overcome his addiction by saying, essentially, "God, help me!" He found other alcoholics in a similar position, and through an organized, non-judgmental support system, they overcame their addiction by realizing that "God" (a higher power, spirit, force, or intelligence) *helps those who help themselves.* In other words, you have to want the help. This is the premise of Alcoholics Anonymous—the most successful recovery program for addicts that exists.

People with other addictions follow much the same program, adapting "The 12 Steps and 12 Traditions," the founding literature for Alcoholics Anonymous, to their particular addiction. Overeaters Anonymous substitutes the phrase "compulsive overeater" for "alcoholic" and the word "food" for "alcohol." The "12 Traditions" in every 12-step program make up a code of conduct, and the theme of all these programs is best expressed through the "Serenity Prayer," the first line being "God, grant me the serenity to accept the things I cannot change; courage to change the things I can; and wisdom to know the difference." In other words, you can't take back the food you ate yesterday or last year, but you can control the food you eat today.

For more on Overeaters Anonymous, visit **www.overeatersanonymous.org**.

Bulimia

Some women feel so much guilt over enjoying and indulging in food that they develop a complex binging/purging behaviour known as *bulimia nervosa* ("hunger like an ox due to mental disorder"). Women will purge after a binging episode by inducing vomiting, over-exercising, or abusing laxatives and diuretics.

> I have only vague memories of eating a meal and allowing myself to be "filled up"— you know—that feeling of warmth and satisfaction after a good meal. Sometimes I wish I could get it back, but I can't allow myself that satisfaction. One day in particular stands out in my mind. I wandered into a bakery after a very stressful day and saw this huge birthday cake. I wanted it, but I was too ashamed to buy it for myself. I told the baker it was for my mother and waited while they wrote on the cake "Happy Birthday Mom." They carefully wrapped it in a box for me. I took it home and consumed the entire cake in about an hour. Then I began to panic. "What have I done?" I kept asking myself. I made myself "do the deed" but I had to throw up several times that night to feel as though the cake was no longer a part of me. Knowing I'd wanted something that large and sinful to go inside me in the first place was a terrifying reality to face; but getting it out consumed more energy than I had. I was so drained and exhausted from the vomiting, I felt I should eat something, but I didn't want to destroy all my hard work and effort. But I was so tired, I thought maybe I could have just some vegetables. Then I had to have dip and vegetables. Then, chips, dip, and vegetables. Then I made pasta, and the cooking and eating went on all night. I called in sick the next morning so I could get everything I ate out of me. My eating and vomiting actually consumed my time and my life for years.

I came to realize much later that the binge/purge pattern I had developed was my way of avoiding life. As sick as it was, it was safer to occupy my time with my bulimia than go out into the world.

Bulimia is also often related to body image. A woman will resort to binging and purging or to not eating (*anorexia nervosa*) in her attempt to control her body size and shape. Many experts see eating disorders as addictions to perfection; the sense of control the eating-disordered woman gains through this behaviour is the drug. Chapter 6 explores bulimia in greater depth.

Not Eating

In times of stress, or at times when they feel that their lives are out of control, women may use food refusal (anorexia nervosa) as a way to regain control in their lives. In anorexia, the person's emotional and sensual desires are channelled through food. These desires are so great that the anorexic fears that once she begins to eat she'll never stop, since her appetite/desire knows no natural boundaries. The fear of food drives the disease.

Anorexics can become martyrs in their refusal of food, feeling more in touch with their lives and their bodies through the suffering that comes with starvation. For more on anorexia, see Chapter 6.

Abusing Drugs

Women will often turn to prescription or illegal drugs to self-medicate for stress. There is a strong relationship between drug addiction and women becoming accustomed to being "tossed" pills by doctors for social problems. In other words, the medical system must take responsibility for encouraging women to run to drugs for help. Too often, women are called addicts—and made to feel as though they are completely to blame for their addiction—when it is their own doctors who helped to addict them in the first place. This is especially true with prescription drug abuse. (Pick up a copy of *Valley of the Dolls*, the classic 1967 pulp-fiction bestseller that exposed the real story of how women under extreme stress get addicted to prescription drugs. Or, try a biography of Judy Garland for a classic story of doctor-caused, or "iatrogenic," drug addiction.)

Prescription Drugs

One of the most notoriously abused prescription drugs in the United States is OxyContin. This drug is widely prescribed for cancer pain or other chronic pain, and is equivalent to heroin in its effects. OxyContin gets into the hands of people who don't need it when doctors, acting unethically, prescribe it to anyone who asks (here, the doctor is basically the "dealer"), or when the prescription holder sells or gives pills to friends or family members. In these latter cases, doctors may become suspicious of the frequent prescription renewals and intervene, or they may just look the other way, in effect behaving as unethically as doctors who needlessly prescribe the drug. Patients may fake pain in order to get a prescription, a tactic doctors may or may not be wise to.

The prescription drugs most usually abused by women are much milder than OxyContin—for example, strong codeine medications, tranquilizers, or Valium, all readily prescribed by doctors for headaches and so on. Women often share drug prescriptions with girlfriends, creating a large pool of Rx concoctions as a sort of "women helping women" type of operation. Legal problems aside, this is not good for you for all the obvious reasons you may know about: the body will require more of the drug over time as it becomes used to it; you may suffer from withdrawal symptoms; all of these drugs have strong side-effects (these can be reviewed in the *Compendium of Pharmaceuticals and Specialties*, located in libraries and online); the long-term use of these drugs can wreak havoc on your liver, the organ through which all medications must be filtered.

Prescription drug dependence is not as widely discussed as illegal drug dependence, and for that reason, many women continue this habit for years without seeking help. Elizabeth Taylor was one of the first women to be open about her prescription drug dependence; she had been struggling with back pain and chronic pain for years, and was unable to get through a day without several prescription drugs. She finally checked herself into a drug treatment program to wean herself off the drugs. Prescription drug abuse usually starts as a temporary solution for a real stress-related problem: headaches, anxiety, back pain, and so forth. The addiction becomes established when the person develops a physical dependence on the drug; the pattern is much as it is for rebound headaches (see Chapter 1).

Illegal Drugs

Woman under stress may turn to cocaine, marijuana, or harsher substances for the same reasons they turn to alcohol. These drugs are "enablers"; they make women feel more powerful and more able to express themselves. One of the emerging patterns in research on women and addiction is that women tend to seek out pleasure drugs, such as cocaine, Ecstasy (also spelled "XTC"), and MDMA (3,4-methylenedioxymethamphetamine, similar in structure to the hallucinogenic drug mescaline).

For a lot of women, taking a drug that heightens pleasure is their first completely self-indulgent experience with pleasure. It is something they can do that is "just for them." When women are denied permission to pursue pleasure on their own, drugs can become their "pleasure enabler." Pleasure drugs aggravate both the physical and emotional signs of stress.

When you smoke marijuana, for example, the amount of tar you inhale and the level of carbon monoxide you absorb is three to five times greater than the levels inhaled by regular tobacco smokers. Marijuana can also increase your heart rate and blood pressure, especially when it's mixed with cocaine. Problems with memory and learning; distorted perceptions; difficulty in thinking and in solving problems; loss of coordination; increased anxiety or panic attacks—all these are common side-effects of regular marijuana use.

The health risks of Ecstasy, cocaine, and crack ("crack" is the street name given to cocaine that has been processed from cocaine hydrochloride to a free base for smoking, a process that produces a crackling sound) are huge: *death from an overdose or a drug reaction is your biggest risk.*

Ecstasy makes the user feel positive, loving and empathetic, totally relaxed and calm. It also suppresses the need to eat, drink, or sleep, enabling users to endure long periods of partying or wild behaviour. It is a classic weekend drug and became popular among the teens and university students who attended all-night raves. Ecstasy is used by older adults, too, not just young adults. The range of side-effects include confusion, depression, sleep problems, anxiety, and paranoia during, and sometimes weeks after, taking the drug. Physical effects include nausea, blurred vision, faintness, and chills or sweating. Increases in heart rate and blood pressure are special risks for people with circulatory or heart disease, and these side-effects can be aggravated if they're on estrogen-containing drugs such as the Pill. Ecstasy is not as addictive as cocaine or heroin, but it takes only one bad reaction to kill you—especially if you overdose. Ecstasy is illegal for a reason: seizures and loss of consciousness are frequently reported side-effects.

Cocaine carries a deadly health risk: because it constricts blood vessels and greatly increases your heart rate and blood pressure, it can cause stroke and heart attack. Cocaine has several immediate effects: euphoria, mental clarity, and reduced fatigue. You feel hyper and full of energy. The high produced from snorting cocaine may last 15 to 30 minutes, while the high from smoking it may last 5 to 10 minutes. Sudden death from cocaine is common, and it's impossible to tell who is more likely to be killed by it, mainly because of problems having to do with product purity or dosage calculation. High doses of cocaine or prolonged use can cause paranoia, particularly if the cocaine is used with crack. Once you're addicted, breaking the habit can cause very severe depression. Snorting for prolonged periods of time can ruin the mucus membrane of the nose and cause the nasal septum to collapse. Most cocaine deaths are from sudden heart attacks or seizures. Mixing cocaine with alcohol produces a separate substance in the body, "cocaethylene." This substance greatly intensifies the effects of cocaine and increases the risk of death from heart attack.

For more information about treatment for drug addiction, see the following websites:

- **narcononcenter.com**
- **cocaineaddiction.com**
- **heroinaddiction.com**
- **marijuanaaddiction.com**
- **methaddiction.com**
- **addiction2.com**
- **stopaddiction.com**

Anything that gives you a euphoric feeling, a rush, or a high counts as an addiction risk, and its use can go out of control in times of stress. The two most common non-drug–related addictions for women are shopping and gambling; both aggravate financial stress, and for that reason I discuss them in Chapter 5. Many women have romance or sex addictions (these are distinct, by the way); these are symptoms of serious relationship problems—even with oneself—which will be discussed in more depth in Chapter 4.

PART *two*

STRESS CAUSES

Now that the signs and symptoms of stress have been explained, this section explores the chief causes of stress for women.

4 FAMILY LIFE, THE SECOND SHIFT, AND RELATIONSHIPS

The majority of women identify family life and relationships as their chief causes of stress. Married women who are employed report that their stress stems from feeling torn between working and being mothers. No woman believes she can perform both roles to her satisfaction, and that creates a great deal of inner turmoil. Child care in North America is in crisis, leaving most women with few choices.

Mothering duties are also distinct from housework; in all studies and surveys of healthy heterosexual relationships, women do the majority of the household chores, even when they are with supportive partners. The mothering, combined with the housework, is why the terms "second shift," "double duty," and "Supermom" have entered into our vernacular in the last 10 years. The second shift can badly damage relationships, leading to divorce or separation. Women who are tired of the second shift either leave their jobs and become stay-at-home moms or leave their partners when they realize that Mr. Supportive Husband is not supportive. Most women never imagine that *they* will become trapped in this classic dilemma, but then they bring home the baby and find themselves living the life they thought was extinct: the 1950s suburban housewife, but with 21st-century pressures. Many women who make the decision to stay home are stressed by "under-challenge" and boredom in their new role as mother, yet feel tremendous guilt over wanting "more from life." Others find staying at home very rewarding, but in recent years, the "happy homemaker" role has been splashed over so many magazines that those who aren't happy at home feel they are bad people.

Single working mothers are the most stressed: they do everything. They have to find suitable child care, work, and go home to the second shift with no help or support. Many women are single mothers by choice: they left troubled or violent relationships or they became mothers with the aid of a friend's sperm or a sperm bank. Women who are single mothers by chance may have been abandoned by their partner or had no choice but to leave the relationship themselves. More common these days than 10 years ago are women in their 30s and 40s who've been widowed due to increasing rates of cancer in young adults, random accidents, and, of course, violence and terrorism.

Single women without children also report that their relationships (or lack thereof) are the main source of their stress. Single women "by chance"—meaning that they are single because they have not found a suitable life partner—find relationships, the dating scene, and the continuous waiting or watching for Mr. Right extremely stressful. Many single women are in unsatisfying and unfulfilling relationships, or find themselves wandering in relationship purgatory, going from one relationship to the next in an endless stream of "serial romances" and repeated patterns.

Caregiving is another huge source of stress for women. Women are the ones in our society who wind up caring for aging parents and children with special needs, without being paid for their work. The appalling lack of child care is equal to the appalling lack of eldercare. Many women cope with both problems. One director of an eldercare facility in California told me: "In the U.S. we are quietly exterminating our elderly because no one can afford to put their parents in facilities, and the hospitals won't take them. They are left to die." Most women in Canada see the same kind of mass "eldercide" taking place. And it makes them physically and emotionally sick.

This chapter looks at all of these issues. It exposes relationship myths that keep many women unhappy. It also validates your feeling that "you're not crazy, the world is." Many women are unaware of the bigger picture behind their limited choices: women who experience the feeling that their options are "collapsing" are also experiencing a world that was not built for, or was not meant to accommodate, mothers, children, or vulnerable people like the elderly and disabled. Many women also don't realize that the 1970s definition of feminism (still prevalent) doesn't accommodate mothers and children, which further traps women. Naomi Wolf, renowned feminist and author, examines the social problems of "motherhood" in her book *Misconceptions*. Wolf reveals that she was shocked to discover that she has been living the life Betty Friedan described in *The Feminine Mystique*, the groundbreaking feminist manifesto published in 1963 that opened with the following words.

The problem lay buried, unspoken, for many years in the minds of American women. It was a strange stirring, a sense of dissatisfaction, a yearning that women suffered in the middle of the twentieth century in the United States. Each suburban wife struggled with it alone. As she made the beds, shopped for groceries, matched slipcover material, ate peanut butter sandwiches with her children, chauffeured Cub Scouts and Brownies, lay beside her husband at night—she was afraid to ask even of herself the silent question—"Is this all?" (Friedan, *The Feminine Mystique*, 15)

Wolf reminds us in *Misconceptions* that nothing much has changed:

My life as a mother had become just what I feared … I experienced a tightening of the world's circumference; I *was* chained to the couch nursing; I *was* stunned with fatigue … I had become all the things I was most afraid I would be. Also, we had moved to the suburbs … I was asked to be a guest at a feminist organization's dinner and had to decline because the event had no child care—no one to hold a baby on her lap in the twenty minutes for which I was asked to speak … my baby was seen [by Wolf's peers] as my awkward living handbag. (Wolf, *Misconceptions*, 209–10)

The Mother Load

When women make the transition into motherhood, the stress can be incapacitating as they cope with postpartum life (fatigue, not getting out, and the demands of a new baby), all the while struggling with the dilemma of whether or not to return to work. If they don't return to work, they feel judged by other working colleagues and fear facing that terrible question "What do you do all day?" If they do return to work, they must cope with the schizophrenic work/home existence, as well as with guilt over leaving their child each morning. Then there is that "other" relationship—the one with the father. Housework issues, competing work demands, and a host of problems can ensue when Junior arrives. The "mother load" is the source of much stress for women.

The Postpartum Period

Most women are unprepared for the life they begin to lead after the baby is brought home from the hospital. The research on this subject yields the same results over and over again: women feel stressed, unprepared, isolated, and depressed, to varying degrees, within the first year of having a baby. In one alarming study of 1,400 American couples, 70 percent of the couples reported that, following the birth of a baby, their marriage had worsened to the point where both the father and mother were unhappy. Eighty percent of women after delivery experience the "blues"; one in four first-time mothers will go on to develop full-blown depression.

> A [North American] woman's main source of postpartum support, her husband, typically returns to work in a culture without mandated or paid parental leave, two weeks postpartum—exactly when the new mother's supposed to be feeling the lift from the "blues." But the combination of the husband returning to work, the sleepless nights, the lingering effects of hormonal plunge, the aching body and demand to single-handedly care for a new baby, can send many women into a downward spiral. (Wolf, *Misconceptions,* 217)

In many cultures—China, Japan, Guatemala, and the Caribbean, for example—new mothers are surrounded with support from their extended family and from other women in their community; they are not expected to do anything very much beyond breastfeeding in the first six weeks after delivery. Most North American women are left alone with a newborn, and experts on postpartum depression believe that this is one of the leading contributing factors in postpartum stress and depression. Not only are families separated by great distances, but there is no extended-family model in North America, since we "warehouse" our elderly. Eighty-seven percent of women take time off from their full-time job to care for a new baby. In Canada, employment insurance (EI) provides up to 15 weeks of maternity benefits and 35 weeks of parental benefits at 55 percent of claimants' insurable earnings to a maximum of $413 a week. This adds up to a minimum of 50 weeks of paid maternity leave, but combined with sick leave, most employed women can take 52 weeks of paid maternity leave.

Postpartum depression occurs in all classes of women. In late July 2000, 37-year-old Suzanne Killinger-Johnson, physician and psychotherapist, daughter of a renowned psychologist, wife of a psychiatrist, and the new mother of a six-month-old son, Cuyler, jumped in front of a Toronto subway, her baby in her arms. Cuyler was killed instantly. Suzanne died, too, after lying unconscious in a Toronto hospital for a few days. Her 1999 silver Mercedes sport-utility vehicle was parked in the driveway entrance to a nearby supermarket. The episode shook the country. The media began reporting on postpartum depression (Suzanne was apparently being treated for this problem). But the clinical definitions of postpartum depression did not answer the question "Why? What *really* happened here?" The answer is that mothers do not have the social and psychological support they ought to have, and this can lead to devastating consequences.

Postpartum depression affects between 10 and 15 percent of the overall postpartum population, which translates into about half a million women each year. This depression can begin at any time after delivery, from the first few hours to a few weeks later. The symptoms include sadness, mood changes, lack of energy, loss of interest, change in appetite, fatigue, guilt, self-loathing, suicidal thoughts, poor concentration, and weak memory. The women most at risk are those who have suffered from episodes of depression prior to pregnancy and those who lack a good support system at home—the latter, according to Naomi Wolf, constitute almost all women in North America.

The "Is Working Worth It?" Question

About ten years ago, I remember seeing this messy woman at Baskin-Robbins totally lose it in public while she was trying to get her whiney, bratty kid to decide what flavour of ice cream he wanted. She started out calm—"Do you want chocolate … or something with fruit …?" The kid was impossible. She ended up screaming: "That's it—no ice cream. You can't behave, we're leaving!" The kid hit her; she smacked him across the face. It was awful, embarrassing, and left me vowing I would never, never become that woman. A few months ago, I was in Loblaws with my four-year-old and two-year-old. They had both just gotten over the chicken pox. My nanny never had the chicken pox, and so I'd let her off work. I called in sick to my office (I'm a travel agent) and stayed home with my children. My boss was not pleased, but I had little choice—my husband was working long hours and was not around to help. (He's an executive and makes a lot more money than I do!) We were out of apple juice and "Goldfish"—everything that mattered to toddlers. So I dragged the gang to Loblaws while I raced around trying to get everything. One of the kids threw up in the aisle. I tore open a toilet paper package and tried to clean it up. Finally, we made it to the checkout aisle—but it was not "candy-free." My four-year-old wanted chocolate, and I just screamed at him: "No chocolate!! Just keep quiet!" Then I noticed that two young women were staring at me, laughing. I realized, at that point, that I had become the "Ice Cream Mom"—that horrible woman I swore I would never become. And on top of "losing it" with my child, I hadn't showered in two days and my hair was greasy. I felt, in that moment, that nothing was working. I can't do both things, I thought. I can't DO THIS anymore. That night, I went home and made a list of the pros and cons of continuing to work. I left my job the next week. It was just too much and not worth it.

Women report in numerous studies that they want to be home with their children but feel they must work to make ends meet. There is a false belief that wanting to be with your child—what anthropologists and other social scientists note is a biological, primal desire—means that you are not a "feminist." Danielle Crittenden, in her book *What Our Mothers Didn't Tell Us,* actually blames feminism for the Superwoman myth. Crittenden argues that no woman can successfully balance career and family; yet those who try, and inevitably fail, are made to feel inadequate—they feel like "bad feminists."

Unfortunately, there exist poor definitions of feminism that assert that women are exactly the same as men and require no special treatment. This is the "dino-definition" of feminism from the 1970s—what working women cling to in order to have equal pay in the workplace. Most feminist scholars worth their salt will tell you that feminism means exactly the opposite. The *true* definition goes: because women are biologically different, are socialized differently, and are emotionally wired differently (which, most believe, has to do with how we're socialized), feminism means that *the interests of women should be valued just as much as the interests of men.* Therefore, since women are mothers and men are not, the interests of mothers and their children ought to be given equal consideration in our society. But the reality is, they are not. Not even by feminist organizations, as Naomi Wolf tells us in her quote on page 10.

The Real Backlash

Women report feeling as though their "hearts are ripped out" every time they leave their child for the office. The morning "primal scene" for many mothers goes something like this: the toddler child grips her legs, won't let go, and cries uncontrollably and passionately: "Pullleeeze don't go, Mommy." Many women report calling home at least six times daily to check on their children. When their jobs are unfulfilling, they find themselves wishing they were home and feeling that being with their child would bring them more satisfaction than their boring job. This creates a lot of stress. On the other hand, when their job is fulfilling, women not only feel guilty about loving the challenge of their job, they feel that they can't give the job their "emotional all" anymore, the way they once did. This situation creates a lot of stress, too, and was poignantly portrayed in the 1987 film *Baby Boom,* with Diane Keaton, whose J.C. Wyatt character must come to terms with the fact that she cannot devote the 70 hours to her job that she did before a baby entered her life.

Since the 1970s, women have been brainwashed into thinking that they would be happier and more fulfilled if they joined the workforce. See Chapter 5 for a look at exactly how fulfilling the workplace is these days. Many women like their actual work but are made sick with stress by the places they are forced to work in and the people they are forced to work with. Today, the mother who does not work is considered a statistical anomaly. Two-thirds of mothers with children under six work at full-time jobs. A Decima poll revealed that 70 percent of Canadian women would rather stay home with their kids than go to work and put them in daycare. Many women say that they're being driven "mad" by having to wrestle with the pros and cons of working and staying home. This may also have to do with the distribution of child-care responsibilities in the home: according to studies, women do roughly 60 percent of all parenting and child care, while 77 percent of mothers are the ones who stay home with a sick child and 62 percent of mothers are responsible for their children's extracurricular activities. Roughly half of all women surveyed about child care and parenting report that they have no outside help. The time that mothers, on average, spend with their children is just over 50 percent more than the time fathers, on average, spend with their children. And although it does "take a village" to raise a family, over 61 percent of both parents work full time, without the support of traditional networks of neighbourhoods and extended families. Families that survived on one income 20 years ago now require two. Put another way, 7 out of 10 Canadian families with children under the age of seven are two-income families. Yet the distribution of child care and parenting is still woefully uneven.

The Child-Care Dilemma

> I live in an upper-middle-class area in mid-town Toronto. All you see are nannies from the Philippines looking after white children. I interviewed many nannies and couldn't find someone whose English skills were good enough. Finally I found a wonderful woman from the Caribbean who was available. But my neighbours and friends all cautioned me: if you don't have a nanny who is from the Philippines, too, then when your Caribbean nanny takes your daughter to the park, the other nannies won't talk to her and she won't go to the park as often, which means your child won't get out as much. I wound up getting a nanny from the Philippines—just like everyone else.

Every working mother who doesn't have a family member to stay with her preschool child when she goes to work faces the child-care dilemma. The choices are exactly these.

Daycare Centres.

Sometimes, if you're lucky, you'll find that daycare is offered on the workplace premises. This is more rare than common. Good daycare centres exist, but they aren't easy to find and waiting lists are long. The facilities, supervision, and child-care skills vary widely. A lot of daycare centres underpay and exploit their staff, many of whom are immigrant women, and in turn they hate their jobs.

Private Daycare.

Here, daycare is offered in someone's house. Usually, a working mother has decided that by taking in other people's children, she can stay home and be with hers. Not her first choice, not your first choice, but an adequate solution in child-care "la-la land." The supervision varies widely and depends on the number of children taken in.

Nannies.

Most nannies are immigrant women, often with no legal immigrant status, who live in the home of their employer. The work is hard and low-paying, but does not require technical skills or good English, which is why women with no immigrant status are often the only ones interested in the job. At least, the reasoning goes, the kids are home in their own environment. But, your "guilty conscience" tells you, your children are being looked after by someone who is not their mother and who couldn't possibly love them as much as you do. What's more, having a nanny live in your house all the time can affect the interpersonal dynamics between you and your spouse. Some nannies do housework, which solves some problems for working women.

Babysitters.

Most women find it difficult to arrange babysitting schedules because their jobs may not be predictable in terms of stress, hours, etc. Generally, those who go the babysitter route wind up with nannies.

Well, there you are. The four lousy options no woman wants. Then comes the math. Most women calculate what they make and then subtract what they pay for child care as well as all the expenses of just going to and being at work (gas, transit fare, dry-cleaning bills, work clothes, pantyhose, cosmetics, lunches, and purchased snacks at work), factoring in tax considerations. They reason: "If it comes out even, I'll stay home." Women who make substantial salaries find it hard to make the stay-at-home decision; whichever option they choose carries emotional costs. No one wins in this child-care crisis.

Even women with power and status face these options. How many of you remember "Nannygate," a prominent news item in 1993? When newly elected President Bill

Clinton decided to hire a female for the job of attorney general, he couldn't find anyone who didn't have an illegal immigrant for a nanny. Why not? Because the only suitable nannies that working mothers could find came from other countries illegally. The Clinton administration did not want to have a woman with "nanny problems" in the job, but instead of looking into the child-care crisis and exploring why intelligent and capable women lawyers like Zoe Baird had such problems, the administration began screening single women for the job. That's why Janet Reno became the attorney general instead of Zoe Baird.

When the math favours working over staying home, the next dilemma that women face is their boss. They want to have a conversation with their boss about the natural and imperative demands of motherhood, but fearing that this conversation will kill their career, they put it off. Eventually, in as politically correct English as possible, they ask their boss the central question: "How many hours must they work to keep their jobs?" The wheels start spinning. Can they work flex-time? Can they work part time, four days a week, telecommute, job-share—*anything not to work more hours than they spend with their children*. Since these dilemmas spill into the arena of women at work, they are covered in Chapter 5.

The bottom line is that all working mothers have to face the "quit or stay" question. They look to other women for solutions, seeking out cures for the problem that won't go away. Women who quit are resented by women who keep working; they are made to feel by some that they are throwbacks to June Cleaver. Women who keep working are criticized by the quitters, or even by their own families, and are sometimes told that their careers are bad for their families. (This interesting tension can be seen played out on Amazon.com. Check out the readers' reviews of a milestone book called *What's a Smart Girl Like You Doing at Home?* by Linda Burton, Janet Dittmer, and Cheri Loveless. This book validates many women's feelings about choosing to stay home.)

The most disturbing comment on the child-care crisis comes from a babysitter. She tells it like it is from ground zero in middle-class North America:

> The kids are spoiled, materially overindulged. The mother gives them affection when she walks in. What she doesn't give them is time. The kids go home in the afternoon, the sitters are so poorly paid that they have little incentive to turn the TV off. The kids have no imagination, they don't make up stories, the TV has become an emotional substitute ... The kid gives you his measles while you are taking care of him, and the mom and dad won't pay for the days of work you lose when you have to stay home sick. (Quoted in Wolf, *Misconceptions*, 259)

The Supermom Disease

A poignant article by Paula Brook, a former magazine editor, is aptly titled "Supermom Goes Home: I Had It All, and Then I Had Enough." It appeared in a 1996 issue of *Saturday Night* magazine and rings even truer today. This little sample speaks volumes:

> I had cultivated the appearance of a calm executive who'd happily reached her stride, while feeling more like a crazed carousel pony going up and down, round and round, faster and faster, about to come unpinned. In effect, I had discovered the Impostor Syndrome, well before the women's magazines announced it.... I lost the ability to concentrate on a single task for more than ten minutes [and] at home it felt like insanity: I cooked and ate in autopilot, one eye on the clock; my rope was only this long for homework help, and I would edit bedtime stories for brevity; I quit jogging in favour of violent spurts on the Stairmaster; I started looking my age, plus ten; I craved a vacation the day after I got back from one.... We are held up as role models, and thus the mania feeds itself. Once you arrive at superwoman status, it is very hard to renounce the role and accept the blame for the stress and misery it can bring.... Certainly [my husband] and I could survive on one income—sell the house, the sofa, whatever—and I could put some real energy into bringing a pulse back into my home. Make it the kind of home I grew up in, instead of a nicely furnished pit where speeding bodies stop for fuel and sleep. (*Saturday Night* 111, no. 5 [June 1996]: 30–38)

What I call the "Supermom disease" mental health professionals call the "pleasing disease"—a term that frequently graces the covers of magazines such as *Oprah*. Women who feel they are failures because they haven't completed every item on a "to do list," or who feel they can't give themselves permission to relax, feel that way because they are conditioned to nurture and to please. When they can't manage all of the tasks at work and at home, instead of slowing down, many women tend to speed up; they become better at multitasking and take on even more. Many women wind up spending more evenings out than they care to with people who drain them, and they commit themselves to more projects than they can handle, which also drains them, simply because they don't feel they are entitled to take time out for themselves and refuse to do something.

It's been long established that women will go to great lengths to preserve connections and relationships with people. They do this because that's how they're socialized. Women will even do things that go against their moral code or value system to preserve relationships in their work and personal lives. When it comes to their children, women will do just about anything to preserve the relationship. For example, many women report that the "equality" between themselves and their spouses erodes when children enter the picture. When repeated arguments over housework and child care create tension in the spousal relationship, and hence tension for the children, many women will just yield in an instinctual act of family preservation. They conclude that it's easier to just *do* the dishes themselves than waste what little energy they have arguing with their spouse over the ethics surrounding "equality and the dishes." It's easier to say "yes" than "no"—to any task—for almost all working mothers.

This behaviour is operative in the workplace, too. It's easier to volunteer to coordinate the company picnic than to sit in the boardroom for 30 extra minutes waiting for someone else to volunteer (fearing deep down that you'll be perceived as a "bad team player" if *you* don't volunteer). It's easier to say, "Sure I can stay and proof that for you," than to explain that you really need to get home. And so it goes. Most women value being liked over being respected, which again has to do with how women are socialized. Always trying to please other people is a huge source of stress *and* anger. Women have great difficulty expressing their anger, and the result is often depression, which health experts refer to as "anger turned inward." Anger is mobilizing, while repressed anger is immobilizing. The physical and emotional consequences of the stress created by the Supermom disease can wreak havoc on your health.

Women who say "yes" to everything are also trying to avoid the terrible guilt they feel when they can't do everything. Expectations about what women ought to be accomplishing—building an enviable career and a family—create tremendous feelings of guilt. Women realize that both can be done—*but not at the same time!* Guilt is distinct from shame: guilt results when women do not meet their own expectations, while shame comes from when they fail to meet someone else's expectations. Often the guilt and shame blur when it comes to Supermoms. Even women who have made a conscious choice to focus on one thing feel guilt over not working on the other part of their life. In my own case, every family function I attend leaves me feeling like an utter failure because I don't have children and have spent most of my time focusing on my career (for example, writing a book such as this). I know that I cannot do both things, but there is an expectation from others that I ought to be doing both things. On the flip side, friends of mine who have quit their jobs to stay home are criticized for not "working." Few women can avoid feeling guilty for not being all things to all people. Women report continuous feelings of never being good enough, there enough, or focused enough for the many people in their lives. Friends, partners, colleagues, family members are all part of the guilt machine. It seems that women can never spread themselves thin enough to cover all of the people who need them.

Ms. Magazine has reported on how "Celebrity Moms" have helped to keep the Supermom myth alive. When celebrities gush over how "wonderful" motherhood is and magazine articles feature Celebrity Moms who balance the demands of their career and motherhood beautifully, ordinary moms are made to feel that much more guilty for failing to meet all the demands on them. Of course, they also don't have the personal assistants, chefs, workout coaches, and all the other support staff most celebrities employ. Celebrities who work hard at their careers and who are quoted saying things like "All I wanted was a baby" or "Happiness is having a baby" help to keep the myth of motherhood (what sociologists call *pronatalism*) alive. Ordinary women with careers who decide that they cannot also be mothers are made to feel incomplete by these testimonials. *Ms. Magazine* points out that the Celebrity Mom articles began to appear with increasing frequency when there was a dramatic rise in the number of women who worked outside the home while raising small children— circa 1983. Today, it's hard not to find at least one Celebrity Mom on the cover of a woman's magazine, reminding us that we are inadequate.

Housework Issues

Housework contributes to a great deal of stress. It's not the individual chores themselves, but the distribution of housework and the arguments over it that lead to stress. In studies and surveys about housework in the homes of heterosexual couples, roughly 66 percent of women report that they're responsible for cooking and grocery shopping, and that includes meal organization and household budgeting. The only job that falls consistently to the man is household repairs. Men are frequently responsible for car maintenance and repairs as well.

Housework is about power relations within a couple's relationship, not about actual chores. As Naomi Wolf observes in *Misconceptions*, the equality between couples slowly erodes when a baby is born—no matter how egalitarian the relationship was pre-baby. This is partly because women are socialized to preserve relationships, as discussed above. But it is also because women are biologically wired to protect their children. As noted above, when a woman senses that fighting over equality issues will affect the dynamics in the household and possibly harm the baby, she will yield.

Sociologists see the division of housework as a broader metaphor for the way gender roles are organized in our society. Most women do twice as much housework as men. Their relegation to housework reflects the job market overall. Women are routinely selected for domestic kinds of work—cleaning, child care, home care, elder-care, nursing, and secretarial. More men are routinely selected for executive positions in upper-level management than women. Men are even more likely than women to attain positions of status and authority in female-dominated occupations, such as the service sector. This pattern trickles down into the household. The fact that there are still female-dominated jobs gets reflected back to working mothers—even if *their* day jobs are as executives and the man is a nurse! In other words, as long as more women are hired as domestics and more men are hired as managers, women will be viewed as being more suited for domestic work. So what are the so-called female tasks at home? Grocery shopping, laundry, making meals, clean-up after meals, and routine general house cleaning are considered "female" tasks. These are the daily tasks, too. Repairs, maintenance, and lawn work are more sporadic and seasonal.

When full-time jobs for both partners stretch into seven-day workweeks (work is routinely done at home on weekends), the housework issue can become even more problematic and poisonous.

Caregiving

Another kind of "mother load" involves the care of aging mothers, fathers, in-laws, and other relatives. In almost all cases, the woman takes on the role of unpaid care-giver. Frequently she is a working mother herself, trying to balance a job and child care on top of caregiving. Caregiving, understandably, is a major source of stress for women, one that largely goes unrecognized and unacknowledged.

> When my mother became severely impaired as a result of Alzheimer's disease, I had to become her decision maker for everything. I had to find suitable home care, which was impossible. (I would stay with her three nights a week.) I also had to assume control over her finances and estate. I sold her car to prevent her from driving because she frequently would be found lost on the road and had gotten into several fender-benders. When she lost the ability to recognize me, she would say terrible things to me and accuse me of stealing from her. I had to quit my job to manage everything in my life. My mother was the last straw and I began to suffer from panic attacks. When we eventually moved my mother into a long-term–care facility, the stress did not go away, because she was not well cared for. I would find her soiled with her own feces and clearly neglected. I felt so guilty for not being able to care for her myself, yet ashamed that I really did not want to take on the burden. She died from a fall (we think), which caused a brain hemorrhage.

A woman in a caregiving role primarily provides personal care in the home of her family member, helping to groom or clean the person and frequently cleaning parts of the home or arranging for the home to be cleaned by a cleaning person or service. In fact, providing personal care and helping with personal hygiene are usually what is required of a professional caregiver from a home-care agency, but because these tasks are considered undignified work, the jobs usually go to unskilled immigrant women who are happy to have a job and opportunity to be in Canada—much the same the situation we see in child care, discussed earlier in this chapter.

Caregiving inevitably involves emotional strain, which is a major contributor to burnout. Women caregivers are distressed by their family member's predicament and their own helplessness in changing that predicament. The latest figures tell us that 10.3 percent of Canada's 3,795,121 seniors require some form of care in the home. Senior women tend to require care more frequently than senior men because women outlive men, and that means more of them end up living alone in their later years. Currently, 42 percent of women aged 65 and over live alone, as do 34 percent of women aged 65–74 and 57 percent of women aged 85 and older. Even people in the prime of health will some day require care; as people get older and become disabled, they require some form of help. Roughly 9 percent of people aged 65–69 need personal care, but as people age, that figure jumps to 45 percent for people 85 and older. There is moderate tax relief for caregiving in Canada. At the federal level, persons with disabilities or their caregivers may apply for the Medical Expenses Tax Credit. However, the tax relief offered is not enough incentive for most caregivers to give up their job. Thus, they find themselves having to take extended time off work, especially when a family member is dying. Laws have been proposed surrounding "eternity care" that would mirror maternity leave or family leave, but that's as far as it's gone. Today, many women are trapped in an eldercare dilemma that mirrors the child-care dilemma. The stress can be truly nightmarish.

In Canada, non-professional caregivers are responsible for 80–90 percent of the assistance provided to elderly persons in their homes. No national policy addressing family members caring for elderly relatives currently exists. Non-professional care-givers of the elderly are currently saving Canada's health-care system more than $5 billion annually; with greater tax relief, we would save more money and could put it toward staffing and other necessary resources for home care. Taxpayers would have to pay 276,509 full-time employees to do the work of the 2.1 million non-professional caregivers now providing the service.

Women doing unpaid caregiving are also at risk of being abused by the person in their care, a frequent problem with dementia. Elderly women, in particular, can become physically aggressive toward the caregiver—hitting, kicking, biting, throwing or destroying objects. Women often have to prevent the person in their care from injuring themselves. Verbal abuse—insults and put-downs—is common, since all of the frustration of the person requiring care gets directed at their main source of outside contact, usually the caregiver.

Physical injuries related to lifting the person requiring care or other heavy objects also occur. Back pain, muscle strain, and a host of garden-variety injuries are common. The eldercare problem is clearly enormous, but it is one of women's hidden burdens. Most men do not deal with caregiving stress in the same way at all. In families where the man's parent requires care, it is often the female partner who will deliver it.

Relationships

In preparation for writing this section, I took a one-day course on relationships that was aimed at individuals rather than couples. Some people in the course were single and not involved; others were single but involved with Mr. Wrong or with Mr. 50 percent (i.e., he was half what the woman wanted, half what she didn't want). Some individuals were married. I enrolled in the course for "research" reasons (ahem). Although I had intensely explored the subject of relationships for other works, such as *Women and Passion*, I was not satisfied that I understood *why* relationships are so stressful, difficult, and unsatisfying for so many women, and *what*, practically, women could do to turn that around. Nor did I understand what I, personally, needed to do to "attract" that special someone who was going to make my life perfect.

What attracted me to the course was its name: "Creating a Love That Will Last." (Hmmm—creating … at least that gives me some control over my love life, I thought.) The seminar was led by marital therapists David Rubinstein and Louise Dorfman, a husband and wife co-counselling team who head up Couple Enrichment Inc., based in an affluent Toronto suburb—the centre of much marital distress! Dorfman and Rubinstein have been married for 28 years and unabashedly admit that their marriage is hard work. Nobody wanted to hear that relationships were work, but we listened, shared, and learned a few basic things that we were sorry we didn't know when we were 20.

The bottom line is that a lot of the stress in our relationships comes from our own unrealistic expectations of relationships. This isn't our fault; relationships are marketed and sold as the panacea for all our problems. "Find the right man and your life will change overnight" is what most women, deep, *deep* down, believe, even though they may say otherwise. Because of this belief, few women are satisfied with their personal lives. Women not in a relationship feel they have failed in life because they were unable to attract the "right man." Many try to "keep busy" while they wait for Mr. Right to fall from the sky. Many women who are married or involved with a man feel they are just settling for what's available. Women experience continuous stress over their failure to meet the right man and the external world's harsh judgment of their circumstances.

For women carrying the mother load (see earlier), the relationships that may have once fit the mold of perfection are put to the test under the stressful conditions of children, jobs, mortgages, and so on. When the relationship is tested, you learn more about the person you're in a relationship with, and that's where the work begins. But since you're working so hard at your job and in the home, *who wants to work at the relationship?!*

Many women saturate their bookshelves with what I call "Karma 101" books. These are books by authors such as Deepak Chopra or Louise Hay, the books we read at night to burning incense that tell us that when we're evolved enough, and "ready" internally, we will know who the right man is because "it will all be effortless." Money will flow from trees and everything we yearn for will come if we are good people. The relationship course taught me to replace "When it's right, it's effortless" with "The right man is worth the effort." Just like anything else in life.

Most of the people enrolled in the course, including me, were surprised to learn what, exactly, the "work" in a relationship entails. *The work begins with you, not him.* By becoming more "yourself," true to your own value systems and needs, you can determine whether you're with someone who is truly compatible or with someone who only passes as compatible. Table 4.1 will help you identify your shared values or shared ethics, the touchstones in your relationship. It will help you evaluate whether you're discarding someone you shouldn't, or worse, *accepting someone you shouldn't.* "Listening with a third ear" and developing critical thinking skills were among the other useful techniques taught in the relationship course that can also help you evaluate what you are hearing from your partner or a potential partner. Critical thinking is questioning the obvious and not just accepting what people say at face value. According to Dorfman and Rubinstein, "a critical attitude penetrates beneath appearances, stereotypes, and conventional wisdom in order to reach underlying truths … it impels us to look behind the façade."

TABLE 4.1   Shared Values

Shared values or ethics are the foundation upon which relationships are built. This is not a list of qualities but a list of the values you feel you emulate, such as truth, freedom, integrity, honesty, and equality. This is the template for you to create your own shared values list—a list that will help you determine whether your partner or a potential partner "walks his talk."

Negotiable	Non-negotiable
(e.g., religion)	(e.g., truthfulness)

Source: Adapted with permission from Couple Enrichment Inc., September 2001.

People often say they believe in honesty, truth, and all kinds of altruistic values, but when they are not true to themselves, their words may not at all match their actions. When a man tells you that he is single, for example, it could mean that he is involved with someone but lives alone. Being "tricked" by what you see instead of really listening to a person can result in your being with someone who not only does not share your values, but who lied his way into your value system. Women with physically abusive men often find this out in harsh and dangerous ways. Men who are emotional abusers (a subject discussed at great length at **Heartlessbitches.com**) can also lie their way into women's value systems; these men can be exposed if you employ the "third ear" or critical thinking.

What Is a Relationship?

According to Dorfman and Rubinstein, a relationship is a dynamic process between two individuals that has the potential to change and grow as each individual changes and grows. Whereas many people believe that a relationship is something finite that just happens to them, these therapists view a relationship as something that is purposefully created, nurtured, and developed over time. In fact, they see the purpose of a relationship as an opportunity for personal growth and development. Furthermore, they state that if you want to improve the quality of your relationship, you need to begin by looking at yourself.

We each have our own value systems, beliefs, passions, and painful memories. These are the things that make us who we are. The first premise is to be true to ourselves. Another person may enhance our lives, but he or she does not "complete" us. Terms such as "soul mate" and "better half" feed into our belief that we are walking around incomplete. Most of us believe that the relationship we form with someone will be the thing that completes us. The stress of feeling incomplete can have devastating consequences for women, leading to depression and anxiety.

The Prince Isn't Coming

Many women are waiting for the Prince while they share a life with a man who won't do the dishes and clips his toenails in bed. That man is not the Prince, just the "guy they're with" while they wait for the Prince. The guy they're with has problems, you see. He's got flaws, debts, an ex-wife, and more baggage than you could fit into your overhead compartments. So the entire time they're with this other guy they think they're just settling for second best. He's the guy they bring to company Christmas parties and weddings, but secretly, they yearn for that Prince. (In my personal fantasy, the Prince is that "bookstore guy"—that *fabulous guy* that some women always seem to meet in bookstores.) While they wait for the Prince, their lives can pass them by. The book *Flying Solo*, by Dr. Carol Anderson and Susan Stewart, is based on interviews with dozens of single and re-singled women. It reveals that a big part of living well as a single woman is to stop waiting for the Prince or, as the authors put it, "to give up the Dream." The Dream, or the Prince, is what creates stress for women. Realizing that the Prince isn't coming or that the Dream is an illusion is what releases us from the prison of unreal expectations.

The Frog in a Prince's Clothing

Many of us *thought* we met the Prince; but we kissed him and went into shock when he turned out to be a frog. What I call "the frog in a Prince's clothing" is a common problem that traps countless women. A good example of such a person is a doctor. Doctors are assigned all kinds of superior qualities because they are in a caring profession. The doctor may tirelessly attend to his patients and give the impression that he is a good person, dedicated, honest, loyal, and so on. But the reality may be the opposite. He may be uncaring and selfish; in fact, his motives for taking on a caring role may have more to do with ensuring that he passes for a certain kind of person than with any desire to help people. Frogs come with all kinds of degrees and credentials. Frogs are usually charming and handsome, and they're frequently emotional abusers. By returning to the shared values exercise in Table 4.1, you can learn to catch these frogs before they catch you!

Negative Relationships

Negative relationships result when we are not true to ourselves, and the resulting stress is unfathomable. We can become so drugged by our wishful thinking that we fall into an endless pattern of relationships with facades. Women are particularly vulnerable to being untrue to themselves because they are socialized to please and not to express anger unless it's in the interest of someone, or something, else: a child, a partner, or a cause. Many women turn anger inward, and it manifests as depression. When this doesn't happen, the anger becomes misdirected and confused, spawning all kinds of negative behaviour and relationships. For most women, anger is *rarely* expressed in "normal" or "acceptable" ways. It usually comes out inappropriately: masked and twisted. Common manifestations of women's anger include:

- **Depression.** Depression in women is commonly understood as anger turned inward. As noted earlier, anger is mobilizing, while depression is immobilizing.
- **Eating disorders.** These are discussed in Chapters 3 and 6.
- **Self-harm.** Self-harm is a broad category that includes harmful addictions, harmful relationships, suicide attempts, self-mutilation, self-destructive or self-sabotaging behaviour.
- **Harming others.** Harming others is another broad category and includes petty crimes such as theft, "vexatious" lies (lies that deliberately hurt versus white lies), harassment (stalking, repeated phone calls or e-mails), violence against children (women's powerlessness can be turned against those with even less power—their children), heinous crimes (murder or extreme violence against others).

Women can form passive-aggressive relationships with both men and women. For example, a woman I know deliberately ends all her relationships by setting up inappropriate conflicts that she refuses to resolve. A missed appointment, for example, might be met with an e-mail accusing the appointment misser of "betraying her" or "ruining her life." She uses e-mail and voice mail to lash out at those who have "disappointed her" (and it doesn't take much!). But then she'll not return the calls (she screens them) or e-mails from the people on the receiving end of her earlier communications when they try to resolve the conflict; this often leads them to becoming enraged. As a result, she's attracted a string of unhealthy obsessive males into her life who try to get even with her. She's been the victim of obscene calls, the recipient of dead animals and flowers, and, oddly, the object of desire for men who secretly thrive on the conflict. This woman admitted to me that she had learned to dodge conflict in childhood: "When my father wanted to hurt me, he wouldn't beat me; he would beat my dog."

Why We Can't Get Angry

Because women grow up in this society in a subordinate role, they can develop an inner belief system that makes it difficult to express anger. Many women believe the following:

1. I am weak. If I express my anger, I'll be overpowered.

2. I am dependent. If I express my anger, I may disrupt my lifestyle.

3. I have no right to feel anger. If I express my anger, I won't be liked or loved as much. (This belief is an extension of feelings of low self-worth and -esteem.)

4. I want people to think I'm nice. I don't want to be labelled a "bitch" or a "nag" or "bitter." (This belief stems from negative stereotypes associated with angry women.)

Women suffer when they feel they are disconnected from the world around them. The anger they feel in consequence may threaten to sever their relationships, and so they may go to great lengths to mask it. Many women rank having a relationship more valuable than having a self. As a result, terms such as *de-selfing* and *silencing of the self* are used in academic literature that focuses on women and anger.

De-selfing, or silencing of the self, means that you're putting your whole value system (what you think, want, etc.) "up for sale" in order to keep the peace in your relationships. The flip side is that when you do this long enough, you become very angry. De-selfing is considered to be at the root of most women's inability to express anger.

> When I first got involved with Dick, he was up front about his drug dealing, which he softened by saying he was just a nice guy "helping out some friends." Even though I felt it was wrong, I never said anything. I didn't want to make him angry, and I was willing to put up with it in order to keep him. One day, he took me with him on a deal (he was selling Ecstasy or "E"). As he drove to the buyer's house, I remember getting very angry, to the point of just seething. I stopped talking and told him that I would wait in the car. He kept asking me if I was mad; he kept trying to find out why I wouldn't talk. I just kept saying, "Nothing; it's nothing." A few months later, he asked me if I would lie for him and say he was with me when he wasn't. I asked him for details, but he wouldn't disclose them. When I said I wouldn't, he accused me of being unfaithful and betraying him. The next morning, I called a taxi and had the driver help me move all of my things out of Dick's place. I went to a girlfriend's. I just left Dick without saying goodbye … without an explanation. It was easier. But then I felt really guilty and worried that he wouldn't love me anymore.

Even when we are justified in feeling anger, we feel guilt. Harriet Lerner, author of *The Dance of Anger*, writes:

> "See no evil, hear no evil, speak no evil" becomes the unconscious rule for those of us who must deny the awareness and expression of our anger. The "evil" that we must avoid includes any number of thoughts, feelings, and actions that might bring us into open conflict, or even disagreement, with important others. To obey this rule, we must become sleepwalkers. We must not see clearly, think precisely, or

remember freely. The amount of creative, intellectual, and sexual energy that is trapped by this need to express anger and remain unaware of its sources is simply incalculable. (Lerner, *Dance of Anger*, 7, 8)

Fatal Attractions and Domestic Violence

According to the most recent Statistics Canada report, one out of four women is being assaulted by a husband or live-in partner. Eighty percent of Aboriginal women have experienced family violence. Domestic violence frequently begins when a woman becomes pregnant, or it escalates as a result of the pregnancy. The abuser perceives a woman's vulnerability as an opportunity to assume more control. De-selfing is frequently the reason a woman stays in an abusive or violent situation. Many women have openly said that they are attracted to angry men because they can't express their own anger. The abuser, studies show, displays a very predictable pattern of behaviour: he swings from long periods of Mr. Wonderful, where he's attentive, romantic, and very sexually satisfying, to periods (sometimes brief, sometimes long) of Mr. Terrible, where he's violent, angry, abusive, and controlling, and displays terrible jealousy and rage. With each reappearance of Mr. Wonderful, the "make-up sex" becomes more intense.

Study after study on domestic violence shows that women in violent relationships come from all kinds of backgrounds, from nurturing to abusive. Women in these relationships can be highly educated, in professions such as medicine, the law, and education; they can also be poorly educated, according to most stereotypes. But it is the women with less education and money who, ironically, have more social support systems in place to allow them to leave. Women with higher education and/or more money tend to stay in these relationships much longer because they are afraid to admit what's going on in their house.

> To outsiders, our marriage looked ideal, and at first it was idyllic. I thought Barry was the most wonderful man I could hope for, and our physical relationship was incredible. Things started to turn when we went into our fifth year of marriage. Barry insisted that I give up my own bank account and deposit my paycheck into his, so we could live as a "family" not as "roommates." He then started to question my requests for money—especially when it was for personal needs such as clothing or getting my hair done. I walked around looking like I was living on welfare half the time. Then Barry would turn around, give me a credit card and carte blanche on what I could spend, but when I came home with new things, he would question my taste and tell me certain things were ugly or "not sexy at all." He would begin to fly

into rages over small things. He never beat me up, but he would grab me, shove me, and most frequently break things around the house that I cared about, like my grandmother's china. This behaviour would go on for a few weeks and then the old Barry would return. He would take me out and we would celebrate the "return." I once suggested that he may be manic-depressive and should perhaps get some help, but that only triggered another rage: "If I'm manic-depressive, it's because of YOU ... YOU made me like this." I began to feel so much shame and embarrassment over my marriage and what it had become that I stopped seeing my friends. I just withdrew and told them "family illness" lies. I said my mother was having surgery; my father was ill; I had chronic fatigue, bronchitis, and things like that.

The typical pattern in domestic abuse is for the abuser to begin to establish control over the woman through verbal put-downs. By the time battering begins, the woman feels so degraded and helpless that she doesn't have the emotional strength to leave.

Gloria Steinem maintains that the more incomplete a woman feels (because of low self-esteem), the more needy she becomes for male approval. She projects all of her missing qualities onto the man. Abuse is perpetuated by the woman's need for this approval and the man's need to prove he's *better*. The projections can lead to other negative patterns, such as obsessions.

Obsessions

Many women in unsatisfying relationships develop obsessions. Women are also vulnerable to becoming the objects of male obsessions and fantasies, perhaps finding the male attention and flattery irresistible. But because we wander into these situations unconsciously, these relationships can become dangerous and unfulfilling, putting our lives or reputations at risk.

Being obsessed with someone means that you are continuously preoccupied with that person. Obsessions usually arise when a romantic interest goes unrequited. In most cases, you invest the object of your obsession with more than he or she deserves; the obsession is built around fantasy and your own need for fulfilment. Your obsession serves to distract you from the more important issues in your life or root causes of your unfulfilment. Women who become obsessed are usually disengaged from their own lives; they may be in unfulfilling marriages or jobs, and they obsess as a way to escape. Obsessions leave women so caught up with someone else's life that they forget about living their own.

> Josh and I were just friends, but I longed for more and wondered if he felt the same way about me as I did about him. I would spend hours analyzing his e-mails, look-

ing for hints of romantic subtext. If he signed off with a "take care" one day instead of a "cheers" I would think for hours and hours about why he carefully chose to deviate from one "sign off" over another. Why was he inserting a happy face at a certain point in the e-mail versus another point? I would save his voice messages and play them back, over and over, looking for "clues" of his interest in me. I would then spend hours crafting e-mails to him, taking my time to carefully word things so he wouldn't "guess" how I felt. When I would send an e-mail, I would check every 10 minutes for a response and would be devastated if I didn't get one right away or elated when it would arrive. This is how I spent my time for months. I would apparently talk about Josh all the time to my friends; I would take every opportunity to insert his name into conversations. If he tentatively suggested we go for a beer or something, I would carefully plan my wardrobe for hours—days before we would meet. I never realized how destructive it all was until one day I lost the ability to work.

When obsessions are requited, they become romantic rescues. But because the romance is based in unreality instead of reality, it cannot be sustained and you may begin to look elsewhere for love. In the end, you might fall into a round of romantic obsessions, a condition that experts call love addiction. The term *addiction* refers to an activity or substance that bolsters you in some way, that gives you a high. The desire to get high on romance is what drives people from one relationship to another. The "romantic" is looking for her fantasy, an impossible ideal that is usually hard to find. She manufactures fiction around a person and idealizes him or her. Women have different romantic fantasies than men; women want to be involved and connected, and are looking for long-term satisfaction. Men, on the other hand, are looking for short-term relationships with big "returns"; Sam Keen, author of *The Passionate Life*, points out that this is the appeal of cybersex and pornography. Even the founder of *Ms. Magazine,* Gloria Steinem, is not immune to romantic addiction.

> So I reverted to a primordial skill that I hadn't used since feminism had helped me to make my own life: getting a man to fall in love with me. As many women can testify, this is alarmingly easy, providing you're willing to play down who you are and play up who he wants you to be. (Steinem, *Revolution from Within*, 264)

Experts who write about romance, love, or sex addiction agree that heterosexual women who continuously seek out one romantic encounter after another are looking for rescue in the form of male approval. They are looking for a man to rescue them from their own bad feelings about themselves. Women who are serial sex, love, or romance addicts feel almost frantic without male approval; only in these situations can a woman lose her self-hood (she de-selfs, as discussed earlier) by adopting the man's needs or values as her own.

Draining Relationships

Another kind of negative relationship is one that is draining.

> I'm a freelance journalist who works from home. I frequently spend more than 14 hours a day writing. I started dating this man who was wonderful in a lot of ways but he couldn't seem to understand why I wouldn't drop what I was doing and edit or ghost write his business letters as favours. One day he phoned me and asked me if I could do some inputting for him; when I asked how long the document was, he said, "About 20 pages—but you're a fast typist, right?" I told him to hire a typist; he asked me why I wouldn't do this for him. Didn't he fix my sink? Eventually I told him that I didn't want to be involved, in any way, in his business or work. He never understood why expending my energy on his administrative work created more stress for me; he just told me I was selfish.

Draining relationships can be with siblings, parents, friends, or co-workers—not just partners or lovers. You may also be draining yourself if you feel sapped by the "absence" of an intimate relationship in your life. Here are some useful questions to help you determine whether your stress may be coming from draining circumstances:

- Do you have someone in your life who offers judgment-free emotional support? This would be a person who makes you feel positive about yourself rather than one who points out your flaws or attacks your choices.

- Are there people in your life who drain your energy and reserves? These people always seem to be in crisis and suck up large amounts of "free therapy" time from you but never seem to be there for you. They may also criticize you and make you feel negative and hopeless instead of positive and optimistic.

- Do you have unresolved conflicts with family members or friends? Unresolved feelings can drain our energy and focus, as we tend to obsess over the conflict.

- Do you feel your friends are more acquaintances and that you lack truly intimate friendships?

- Do you feel a void in your life because you don't have a romantic partner?

- Are you in a romantic or sexual relationship that you know isn't good for you but that you can't seem to end?

- Are you in a relationship that compromises your values? (See Table 4.1.)

- Is there someone in your life who continuously breaks commitments or plans so that you're constantly having to reschedule your arrangements with this person?

Relationship Counselling

Even women in good relationships find that they don't have enough time to nurture them. Women report that they frequently live on a completely different schedule than their spouse and may not even have time to talk to him during the day. Couples may not understand how to resolve conflicts, and a relationship can dissolve into what Dorfman and Rubinstein refer to as a "critical atmosphere," in which a partner is demeaned or ridiculed, left to feel that nothing she or he does is good enough. On the other hand, their Couple Enrichment Approach™ encourages a "caring confrontational atmosphere," where the aim is to "raise the level of awareness or consciousness of one's partner" because of the desire to see her or him grow. In practical terms, instead of yelling about housework, partners could point out that when housework isn't shared, it creates inequality, even though both partners may share the value of equality (see Table 4.1). If the following statements ring true, you may benefit from relationship counselling:

1. You and your partner have difficulty resolving conflicts.
2. You and your partner never discuss your relationship.
3. You feel your partner doesn't really know you.
4. You feel you don't really know your partner.
5. You find yourself criticizing your partner all the time.
6. You feel closer to your friends than to your partner.
7. You blame each other or stonewall each other all the time.
8. You feel lonely in your relationship.
9. You're showing symptoms of stress (see chapters 1 and 2).
10. You're self-medicating for the stress you feel about your relationship (see Chapter 3).

5
WORK, MONEY,
AND FINANCES

The workplace is a volatile stress factory for most female employees. Women may be trying to juggle their job with family responsibilities, break the nearly impenetrable "glass ceiling," and cope with sexual harassment or workplace bullying—the latter frequently perpetrated by female co-workers whose powerlessness or vulnerability in their *own* jobs fosters survivor behaviour, where other competent women may be seen as a threat. Agism is another problem: as women age, they are seen as less valuable by their employers, and workplace "restructuring" forces many of them into early retirement when they can't afford it. In 1997 only 25 percent of women aged 65 to 69 received income from a private pension, compared to 50 percent of men in the same age group. Pensions—both private and government—are lower for women. Since all pensions are calculated over lifetime earnings, women who leave the workforce to raise families lose out; women are routinely paid less during their lifetime, too, which reduces their pensions. For example, since the 1970s, job growth for women has been mainly in the poorly paid service sector. Right now, there is a large pool of highly skilled women in their late 50s and early 60s who must work to live but cannot find jobs.

The workplace is unquestionably ghettoized by gender. The professions and sectors that are dominated by women not only tend to pay lower salaries, but offer less decision-making powers on the job. Poor wages and no autonomy create higher levels of chronic stress. Then there are the still male-dominated sectors (e.g., jobs in the executive track) that offer higher salaries, more security, and decision-making powers.

These inequities create further inequities down the road when women approach retirement; as noted above, many receive lower pensions and have less retirement income than men. Currently, many women over 65 are living in poverty.

Some jobs cause trauma, too. Criminal justice personnel, lawyers who fight social injustice, firefighters, ambulance drivers, military personnel, and disaster teams witness horrific scenes each day. Nurses, physicians, caregivers, social workers, and therapists experience vicarious traumatism, meaning that they are traumatized by what they see and hear on the job. Even ordinary jobs can be traumatic when clients are emotionally or physically abusive.

Women dominate the unpaid work sector, known as the *shadow economy* or *invisible work sector*. Statistics Canada defines unpaid work as all household work that could be done by a third party, such as domestic chores, child care, and shopping. Volunteer work is also unpaid and is largely provided by women. Women who spend their lives doing unpaid work are not entitled to any retirement benefits. On a global scale, the United Nations has estimated the value of women's unpaid work to be roughly $11 trillion (U.S), but this doesn't even count in our current economy. That's alarming considering that it is this unpaid work that supports the "market," or traditional, economy. When you add it up, women are responsible for 68 percent of the world's economy but earn only 10 percent of the world's income; furthermore, 70 percent of people living in poverty are women. Clearly, women are not reaping their share of the resources, and that's because their work doesn't count.

Speaking of counting, continuing problems with women and math literacy play into all of this. A large body of research in gender differences in learning and education shows that women develop different skills than men when it comes to solving math problems. Women prefer to use techniques other than just memory retrieval to solve math problems, and this has to do with how they're socialized and their confidence levels. Consequently, there is now an awareness of the need for girls' math classes, taught largely through group work, which we now know can foster greater math literacy. Unfortunately, many women were not taught math properly and dropped this subject early in high school; they've thus been left with terrible phobias around anything that involves math—investment charts, interest rates, percentages, mortgages—and an inability to handle so many of the basic things that are essential for our financial survival. Women with low math literacy also wind up needing men or a third party to make financial decisions for them.

Women may develop spending habits that are incompatible with their incomes. Sometimes this is related to a complex addiction, such as a shopping or gambling addiction. Like other addictions discussed in Chapter 3, spending addictions give women a high that makes them feel better and, in most cases, distracts them from their problems. The character Carrie in the TV show *Sex and the City* spends $500 that she doesn't have on a pair of shoes when she's depressed, adding to a collection that is already mind-boggling. Shopping addictions can put women in serious debt.

Then we have to factor in how loss of a relationship, through divorce, desertion, or death, affects a woman's financial security. Nearly half of all new marriages end in divorce, and one-fourth of all divorced women in North America live at or below the poverty line. Generally, a woman's standard of living falls 27–45 percent within the first year after a divorce, while a man's rises by an average of 10 percent.

All these issues converge, spelling greater financial insecurity, greater debt, and less economic independence for women than for men. Many feminist economists refer to this as *gender economics*.

There is some good news. Given everything against them in the traditional work-place, many women conclude that they might be better off working for themselves. Canada has a higher percentage of women-started businesses than any other country in the world; women make up 50 percent of small business owners, and there are now over one million women entrepreneurs. Furthermore, if banks treated women entre-preneurs in the same way they treat male entrepreneurs, more women than men would be starting up businesses. Roughly 77 percent of all women entrepreneurs, however, are forced to finance their businesses on their personal credit cards. Routinely, Canadian banks practise blatant sexist lending policies in all areas of financing; this practice keeps many women from being able to own property, improve their financial status, and ultimately realize financial independence. Banks infantilize women by forcing them to find male co-signers, many of whose credit ratings may well be more questionable than the woman's. Banks defend their lending policies by saying that they lend equally according to income levels. But because women earn less than men, in many cases do unpaid work, and are often self-employed because of unfair social arrangements in both the workplace and our society, using income as the only standard remains woefully unfair and inadequate, if not unethical.

The upside of women being compelled to finance their business through personal credit cards or personal lenders (family or friends) is that they feel less *chronic stress* because they are controlling their own destinies. On the other hand, women business owners can expect to suffer from *acute stress*, which often comes with the responsi-bility of making decisions. Acute stress is the "good stress" that motivates and chal-lenges us creatively when we feel that our opinions or decisions are valued.

This chapter looks at the story behind the story when it comes to stress caused by work-related issues, money, and finances. It does not offer serious moneymanagement solutions or investment strategies, however. For that kind of information, you might refer to *Balancing Act*, a book by Joanne Thomas Yaccato.

The Same Old Story

I was travelling from Toronto to Vancouver last year with a full-fare ticket, thanks to a last-minute meeting I had to attend. I had to cancel a family wedding in order to make the trip, and so I decided to travel "up" and paid another hundred bucks to upgrade my ticket to business class. It was my first time in business class, and I was struck by the fact that there were no women sitting in this section—except for me. The entire section, which was not filled up at all, comprised white and Asian men. It was a long flight with delays. You could hear babies crying in "cattle class." All I was thinking was that the most comfortable seats were taken up by the people who least needed them, while the mothers travelling with children were forced to sit in cramped quarters; mothers with small babies had to hold the babies on their laps for over five hours. I wondered how many of the mothers in the back were once working women like myself. If anyone says there is no "glass ceiling," just take a walk down the business class aisle on the "red-eye." I was embarrassed to be sitting there, eating my full-course lunch with wine, when so many of my "sisters" were being tossed peanuts as though they were animals. It didn't even feel like Canada; it felt like some Third World country.

It's official: there are exceedingly few women CEOs (chief executive officers) and few women in truly top jobs. In Fortune 500 companies, the number of women in upper-management jobs and on boards of directors remains very small. Most CEOs acknowledge that "it's unfortunate" that so many women must interrupt their careers to have children; they maintain that the low representation of women in the big jobs is not a reflection of bias but of the simple facts of life. Many male CEOs interviewed about the absence of women in CEO positions say things like: "We're hiring many young women as trainees and expect the ratios to change." But, as discussed in Chapter 4, unless there is radical social change in child-care and family arrangements, women will routinely leave their jobs when they have a family. Many CEOs also acknowledge that having a woman on the board of directors "disturbs" the working environment.

The 21st-century workplace is still a hostile place for women. Here are some truths according to Shere Hite's groundbreaking 2000 book *Sex and Business*.

- Fifty-one percent of women with male bosses feel undervalued.
- Male bosses resist promoting valued female employees, even when they're more talented than their male colleagues, because they're afraid of how the male colleagues will respond.
- Male bosses routinely prefer to hire attractive women over unattractive women, yet this does not hold true for the men they hire.
- Women wanting a promotion won't be promoted unless they disclose their desire for a promotion, but when they do, they may be labelled "too aggressive," "unfeminine," or a "bitch."
- Women routinely work harder and demand less than their male colleagues.
- Women can only succeed when they simulate "male" behaviour and must even act like men with women colleagues, establishing hierarchical management styles instead of working collectively.
- Women routinely withhold their opinions or ideas from male colleagues for fear of being demeaned.

The reality is that women feel they can only succeed in the traditional workplace if they act like men or define their working relationships according to male standards. But women are not men; they have been socialized much differently and lead different lives than men. Women report that much of their stress comes from hiding their female lives from their male colleagues—lives that include being a mother and feeling connected to a child and a family.

The Mommy Track

Before I had children of my own, I was critical of female colleagues who openly brought their child-care problems to work. Women who left meetings early to pick up their kids were looked down upon by my male colleagues, and I soon followed suit. Then I started worrying about not making it to the daycare on time. I mean, the children get really upset when you're late. I feel terrible for judging other women all these years.

The biggest irony for working women on the "Mommy Track" is that government policy does not encourage Canadian companies to help working mothers (through job-sharing programs or flexible schedules) because it is now technically illegal for employers to discriminate in any way between their female and male employees. This stems from old battles and outdated definitions of feminism, discussed earlier.

In many companies, childless women with the same education, skills, and job description as men earn the same as men. But once women have children, their salaries radically decline compared to those of men; the men continue in their careers and move up, while the women interrupt their careers and stagnate. Women are routinely "laid off" or told that their jobs have become redundant when they announce they are pregnant. Technically, they cannot be fired. Firing would be outright discrimination against mommies, as a 37-year-old Ottawa bookkeeper, Jennifer Hanson, proved. She received a court-awarded settlement of $20,000 as compensation for being fired by Reform MP David Chatters five days after giving birth to her second daughter in 1996.

Single mothers are especially trapped by their employers' expectation that they will put in the same number of hours as men when they cannot. CBC Television producer Huguette Cyrenne, for example, was left with no choice after her divorce but to resign from the CBC and take a much easier job as a secretary—at a much lower salary.

When single mothers can't afford daycare or nannies, they're often forced to stay home and live on welfare. In many European countries—Belgium, France, and Sweden, for example—child care is considered a community responsibility and is subsidized when women return to work. In Canada it is privatized, just like the airlines, which creates terrible inequities in the workplace. Child-care workers receive the minimum wage when the pay is generous, but that still winds up costing single mothers roughly $465 a week (based on about $8.00/hr. for 55 hours per week—the average amount of child care required each week). This is simply too high a cost for many working mothers.

A sick child, a doctor's appointment for a child, a meeting with teachers—these are responsibilities that can also cause problems for the working woman. On days when their children take them away from work, many women are forced to lie and tell their employer that they themselves are sick and must take the day off.

The outdated "women are the same as men" approach, as opposed to the "women's and men's interests are of *equal value*" approach—the accurate definition of equality—has done a lot of damage in the workplace. Women are afraid to admit that they cannot put in the same hours as men, in the same way. Companies began to realize in the mid-1990s that they were forcing their mothers out. Deloitte & Touche, for example, estimated that they paid roughly $40 million per year in turnover costs because of the loss of talented women who could not balance the pressure to bill long hours against the needs of their children. Although the firm tried offering flexible hours and part-time arrangements, many eligible women declined to take them because of the fear of being regarded "uncommitted" by their peers. What companies are just now starting to realize is that an offer of flex-time and job-sharing to *all* employees, not just "mothers," would be the great equalizer. At the Royal Bank of Canada, 30 percent of the more than 40,000 employees, both men and women, are on some sort of flexible work schedule. Many employees without children work flex-time. (Don't cheer too loudly though: as noted above, all Canadian banks, including the Royal Bank of Canada, routinely deny women credit and financing for mortgages or businesses.)

The problem is that not all companies have broken from the traditional way of doing things; in fact, exceedingly few companies are "family-friendly." *Ms. Magazine* exposed that the often-publicized "great benefits" offered by Fortune 500 companies are not offered to women who work in lower-paid jobs, for example. Many of these companies' family-friendly policies are immediately linked to salaries and offered to only certain segments of the employees within the companies.

Ms. Magazine revealed that Marriott International, for example, was listed as one of the best companies for working mothers; it offered flexible work schedules, hotlines to help employees deal with child-care emergencies, and three on-site child-care centres. When a waitress at the San Francisco Marriott (whose hours are constantly being switched at the last minute) tried flex-time, she was given a bad performance review by her supervisors and told that she needed to work more regular hours. Essentially, workers in entry-level, low-paying, or low-status jobs are not entitled to family-friendly benefits, even though the companies may boast them.

Women report that they are more stressed when they work compressed work weeks or part time, because the amount of work that needs to get done doesn't diminish even though their hours do. Many women feel that they are being paid half their salaries for a full-time job. Many also feel that time away from work can erode their authority or standing in the workplace. Today, a two-income, 65- to 80-hour workweek is the equivalent of a single-income 45-hour workweek of the 1970s. In other words, people are working twice as hard to stay in the same place as they were in the 1970s.

Women Mistreating Other Women

Women mistreating other women is another "same old story" in the traditional workplace, but one that has been under-reported. What generally happens is that some women will take out their misery on other women or will shout at other women in front of male colleagues. Female secretaries may also treat their female bosses with less respect than they would a male boss. Workplace bullying has become a common problem for women, and the bullying is often perpetrated by a women supervisor or co-worker. Bullying is different from sexual harassment (see further on) in that sexual comments are not involved, but like sexual harassment, the bully is trying to control another person through mistreatment.

> When I started working as a junior copywriter in this large agency, I was happy my boss was a woman. But I didn't bargain for being made to cry all the time by the senior copywriter, who was also a woman but was very cold and dismissive of me from day 1. She's always making these quiet put-downs and actually rolls her eyes when I try to contribute ideas at our creative meetings. She looks at other co-workers with these knowing glances as if I'm crazy. She'll also say things like "nice pants" in a sarcastic tone, as though I must look terrible in them or something. Whenever we have to work together, she sits in her office with her feet up on her desk, barely listening to me, while she does her nails. She makes my day a living hell, but if I complain to my boss, I'll just look like I'm weak.

Not all woman bullies are direct; many use passive-aggressive bullying. The bully, for example, may be friendly and open to her "target" face-to-face, but belittle her, gossip about her maliciously, and malign her to colleagues. She often acts as though she has been "wronged" but doesn't know if she should say anything to the boss. She may use half-truths and lies to fabricate terrible stories. This is the most dangerous kind of workplace bullying because the target of the bullying doesn't understand why, suddenly, none of her peers or co-workers are treating her with respect. Sharing private e-mails from the target with others and assigning demeaning tasks to the target are other forms of passive-aggressive bullying.

Another form of bullying is an even more transparent attempt to demean the target. Suddenly the target finds that she's been left out of the loop on important documents or meetings, or has been removed from certain listservs. Women have even been denied their legal rights in the workplace by these type of bullies, not being allowed to have breaks, take sick leave, and so on.

Then there is the commonly reported tantrum-throwing—the clichéd female boss who screams at her target, curses, and is emotionally volatile and explosive.

All of these bullying behaviours stem from old problems in the workplace that make women feel insecure, undervalued, and threatened. Women's unexpressed anger was explored at length in Chapter 4; bullying is another way that unexpressed anger gets manifested in the workplace.

Most women wind up leaving a job where they are bullied because they cannot afford the legal costs of suing their employer. The bullies know that their tactics will get rid of a perceived threat, which is why this problem persists. The Canadian-made series *Beggars and Choosers* (about the goings-on at a large television network in Los Angeles) has a continuing plot line about bullying. One established female executive begins to bully the newly hired female executive in very passive-aggressive ways. The punchline is that the newly hired woman is able to hold her own and manipulates the situation to her advantage—the happy ending the female targets of most bullies never see. They wind up leaving their jobs humiliated, feeling as though the rug was pulled out from underneath them. The situation is all the more painful because it was another woman who pushed them out.

What do male supervisors do about bullying? Frequently, the problem never gets reported because of the Catch-22 involved. The target doesn't want to look like a peer basher, or worse, live up to the cliché that women can't work together. The bully, of course, denies the problem if she's ever confronted. And since the bully is much more familiar with the ins and outs of the corporate culture (the bully is always the "established" employee, while the target is the "new one"), she is able to appear to be the credible voice in the situation.

Sexual Harassment

Shere Hite's research from 2000 reveals that an alarming 76 percent of women report that they have been, or are currently being, sexually harassed. Sexual harassment is not the same thing as sexual banter, on an equal footing, between male and female co-workers. In the classic definition of sexual harassment, a senior worker applies "sexual pressure" (the pressure to perform sex or to begin dating) on a junior worker. The situation could involve a senior female demanding sexual favours from a junior male, but much more commonly it involves a senior male demanding sexual favours from a junior female. What counts as harassment is flirtation in the form of provocative, longing looks; unwanted touching; unwanted kissing; or suggestive or rude comments. The aim in harassment, as in bullying, is to humiliate the target.

When a woman is the target of harassment, she is automatically marginalized and made to feel out of place. Some women are made to feel as though they are "asking" for it. Like the bully, the harasser usually has more solid footing in the organization, so when the harassment is reported, he can more easily escape repercussions or even deny the accusations, putting the onus on the target to prove her allegations.

Flirtation is not the same as harassment, but because it can quickly cross the line, it is discouraged. Nevertheless, flirtation is accepted as a normal, pleasant form of communication between the genders that is not intended to cause harm. Compliments such as "Great haircut!" or "You look nice in that colour" are harmless. They only cross into harassment if they're accompanied by a wink or lewd gesture. Comments such as "Great haircut—I'd like to run my fingers through your hair sometime" or "I'd love to know if you're a real blonde" are harassment. "That's a pretty sweater" or "That's a nice skirt" are compliments or flirtation. "Your tits look really great in that sweater" or "Your ass looks great in that skirt" are examples of harassment—even if you are pleased with remarks like these. A man who respects a woman in the workplace ought not to be commenting on her "tits" or "ass." A man who likes you and wants to get to know you better in a respectful way will most likely avoid any comment that would embarrass or compromise you. (Charm can be an alarm bell, too—see Chapter 4, page 125.) Harassment is meant to cause harm and is unpleasant. If you're in a situation where you are unsure about whether you are being harassed, you probably are. The uncertainty over whether that comment, remark, look, or touch is normal behaviour is a sign that the behaviour is inappropriate—especially if you feel "funny" or compromised as a result.

Harassment and bullying can blur together. A male harasser may not be attracted to a female target, yet he'll make comments that confuse her and make her feel self-conscious about her body. Overweight women commonly suffer this sort of abuse in the workplace. Men have been known to make references to their "big fat ass" or even say outrageous things like "I'd like you to sit on my face and crush me" or "Smother me with those huge tits." The woman knows that the man isn't serious, but she's completely humiliated and sexually objectified nonetheless.

Sexual harassment can lead to a variety of stress-related physical and emotional health problems. These include eating and digestive disturbances as well as excessive weight loss or gain. Anxiety, panic attacks, teeth grinding, insomnia, and nightmares are commonly reported to psychologists who specialize in sexual harassment. Many women develop full-blown episodes of depression, too.

The Glass Ceiling Syndrome

Routinely, women witness their less or equally credentialed male colleagues rise to the top as they stagnate, are made redundant, and are eventually forced out of their jobs. Women begin to see the glass ceiling when they make proposals or suggestions that get dismissed while the same or similar proposals from a male colleague win accolades.

Some shattering of the glass can be heard, however. Carleton Fiorina, for example, was made CEO of Hewlett-Packard in 1999. She was the first female CEO of a Fortune 50 company but only the third woman to make CEO among the Fortune 500 companies. But the reality is still this: half of all the women who work earn less than $25,000 per year.

A Canadian politician provided one of the most interesting shattered-glass stories I know of. Although Kim Campbell became the first woman minister of justice and attorney general, as well as the first woman prime minister of Canada, she became a "fall girl" for Brian Mulroney, whose popularity had plummeted in 1993. Mulroney was determined never to lose an election, and so when one had to be called within a few months, like a good Shakespearean king he plotted his graceful exit. He decided to resign as prime minister and allow a new leader of the Progressive Conservative Party to take his place. By quietly endorsing Campbell, a woman candidate, he allowed himself to appear to be enlightened. Kim Campbell won the Tory leadership race and promptly became Canada's nineteenth prime minister. But she had taken a poisoned chalice! Even so, with scarcely any experience in the difficult role and little time to prove herself or even get a new desk, she called an election just two and a half months later. The election was disastrous. The PCs won only two seats in Parliament, not enough to have official party standing. In this story, an experienced male politician had used the glass ceiling as his escape route. Campbell had inherited Mulroney's campaign staff and was never properly prepared for the campaign trail, which is something even long-standing politicians find gruelling.

Then comes the same old story—Campbell's clothing, hair, makeup, earrings, and marital status (she was referred to as "twice divorced," unlike male counterparts) were more extensively reported than what she said. Campbell made the fatal error, too, of speaking from her heart, rather than speaking from scripts, and for this she was harshly criticized. When, rather than sell them hope, she told voters that the economy would not dramatically improve until the late 1990s, critics felt she was doomed. (It did in fact take until the late 1990s for the economy to improve!) When she acted "like a woman," she was criticized. Had she been more able to don a male persona, she would have been considered successful. The worst was yet to come. In her speech conceding defeat, Campbell joked, "Gee, I'm glad I didn't sell my car," a comment more telling than the public realized. Campbell left Parliament with no pension and an uncertain financial future. For years she relied on lectures to make a living. But all of her male predecessors were made corporate directors. John Turner, whose defeat was even more abject than Campbell's in some ways, got 10 corporate directorships, which spells 10 different paychecks from 10 separate companies. And because all the men had years of experience in Parliament, they all drew healthy pensions. Almost all her male predecessors also went on to earn salaries as part-time lawyers in big law firms. Campbell, also a lawyer, as well as the first woman minister of justice, enjoys none of that. Only recently was she made the Canadian consulate general in Los Angeles, not a plum picking for a woman of so much promise. Campbell's downfall is the sort of thing women in corporations experience all the time. They are frequently "set up" for success and then forced to leave the position for reasons of "creative difference."

Women of colour have an even harder time shattering glass, even when they are in so-called feminist organizations. In 1992, Joanne St. Lewis became the first black executive director of the Women's Legal Education Action Fund (LEAF), a feminist organization that attempts to influence Supreme Court decisions. Eventually, Lewis was forced out of LEAF after enduring repeated questioning of her decisions. The stress was so bad, in fact, that she is reported to have suffered from serious physical ailments as a result.

Women CEOs make half the salary of male CEOs. In the non-profit sector, for example, the average salary in the U.S. for women CEOs was $170,000 compared to $265,000 for men. To add insult to injury, many companies that appear to be woman-owned are actually owned and operated by men. For example, MacDonald Communications Corporation owns and operates *Ms. Magazine*, *Working Mother Magazine*, and *Working Woman Magazine*, and operates the National Association of Female Executives!

For more information about the glass ceiling, visit **www.theglassceiling.com/ glass**. There are many terrible tales to explore, tales that will validate your own experiences with glass ceilings.

Women in Academic or Professional Training

A great deal of stress for women comes from graduate school, where they go through training to become doctors, lawyers, MBAs, or accountants, or where they "upgrade" their credentials in preparation for master's and doctorate degrees. Many women enter university for the first time later in life to obtain undergraduate degrees. In short, many women, in addition to balancing work and family, are balancing work, family, and college or university undergraduate and graduate training programs. Tales of the academic glass ceiling are rampant, as are reports of sexual harassment or bullying of women entering professional schools that used to be male dominated.

Self-employment and Self-financing

When women experience the glass ceiling or other harsh realities of the traditional workplace, many decide to start their own companies and go it alone. In fact, over 650,000 Canadian women are self-employed and the number is growing each year.

More women start their own businesses than men, but women can wander from the glass ceiling to the iron gates when it comes to financing from the banks. As discussed above, banks are much more likely to take a risk with a male entrepreneur than with a female entrepreneur. Although male business owners also complain about financing, more men are granted lines of credit for start-up companies than women. Banking is about relationships. In most banks it is the men who have the final say about credit, and men are more likely to choose to have a financial relationship with a male entrepreneur than with a female entrepreneur. A man is more likely to success-fully access the "gatekeeper" than a woman, since the gatekeeper is usually male.

When you need a loan for anything at a bank, your first point of entry is the personal loan officer/personal banking specialist/personal banking officer; for the purposes of this section, I'll stick to the latter title. These are the people in the small offices who sit down with you and look at your banking portfolio, get all the neces-sary forms, and essentially make you believe that it is with *them* that you have the rela-tionship. But when you leave the bank, these people have to get everything approved by their superiors, and that includes their superiors in the credit department, which is not on location in the bank. The people who make the credit decisions are mostly male. Banks have recently made a point of having several women in personal bank-ing officer positions. Women customers usually get a woman personal banking offi-cer; the banks want women to feel comfortable, and they find that women are less intimidated when they are dealing with another woman. That woman, however, has limited power in her role. Women customers frequently walk away believing they will get their mortgage, line of credit, and so on, only to be told the next day that the "credit department" won't approve the loan application without a co-signer. That means a man with a job, usually. Women also find they are shuffled around within the bank and are unable to access the same services as male customers.

When women entrepreneurs are surveyed about the biggest challenge in starting their business, most rank financing over stress or long hours. Self-employed women also find it next to impossible to get mortgages or other personal loans because lend-ing institutions base self-employed income on net income instead of gross income, which is grossly unfair in most cases. Because child-care dilemmas force so many women out of the traditional workplace (see Chapter 4) and women lack the opportunities for advancement that men enjoy (the glass ceiling syndrome), more women than men are self-employed out of necessity. "Self-employed" has become a euphemism in the banking world for "high risk, poor candidate." Women report being treated like lepers by lenders when they say they are self-employed.

An alarming 1999 study published in *Atlantis* followed two mortgage candidates, with the same income and in the same profession, who applied for an insured mortgage through the Canadian Mortgage and Housing Corporation (CMHC). An insured mortgage means that banks take no risk for the mortgage, and if the mortgage holder defaults, the CMHC pays the bank back the loan. CMHC guidelines stipulate that a certain level of income must be present for the applicant to qualify, but the source of income, gender, or ethnicity of the applicant is not an issue. A calculation of income, minus debt, determines whether you fall within the guidelines. So long as you are not over your debt ratio, you qualify under CMHC guidelines. Two graduate students posed as applicants: one was a single, white male; the other was a single mother. The male was offered a mortgage by several banks at competitive rates, while not one bank or trust company was willing to give the woman a mortgage without a co-signer. The study concluded: "Not only did lenders stereotype, they refused to offer loans that are within CMHC guidelines, thus violating federal and provincial government policy, as well as stated financial institution policies." The CMHC-insured mortgages, however, were designed to end discriminatory lending practices, enabling people with as little as a 5 percent down payment to get a home.

When you consider all of the information discussed in Chapter 4 and "The Same Old Story" section in this chapter, all lenders being equal, women generally have a harder time meeting bank or CMHC income guidelines because they are often forced to leave good incomes to care for their children; they are often abandoned by spouses or forced to leave marriages because of violence or other forms of abuse; and they are forced out of jobs because of the glass ceiling syndrome. In other words, even on a level lending playing field, things are not all that level or equal for women.

Women in Debt and Poverty

Women make up the majority of people living on or below the poverty line. Women in debt put a new spin on poverty. Their poverty is often disguised by seemingly comfortable surroundings, and meanwhile they've "maxxed out" their credit cards to pay the rent in between jobs or contracts, are being harassed by creditors, and are one day away from having their car repossessed. It's also important to note that many women in poverty or debt are also the "hidden homeless," the ones who are not visible on the streets. Untold numbers of women camp out on the couches of friends and relatives, looking for employment or a place to live. For university-educated women, the most common cause of debt and poverty is unemployment, which can breed depression, overspending, and a cycle of hopelessness. Since it can take, on average, three to six months to find another good job, most women don't have the savings to get them through a period of unemployment; instead they incur more debt and often have to give up or downgrade their shelter.

Overall, roughly 3 million Canadians live in poverty, and the majority are women. Two-thirds of food bank users are single mothers, while close to half a million children in this country—most of them in households headed by single mothers—are considered "food insecure" by Statistics Canada. According to the latest National Population Health Survey, half a million Canadians do not have enough money for food.

Leaving a partner who helped to support them or losing a partner through death, desertion, or divorce has a significant impact on a woman's financial status. Women leaving a violent or abusive partner, for example, see a 75 percent drop in income, which affects their ability to find shelter and food. Women over 65 are another impoverished group: because of improper planning, women may not have access to spousal pensions after their husband dies, and women who didn't work in the traditional workforce for long periods or at all receive dismal Canada pensions. Moreover, since women live longer than men, more women than men live with disabling diseases due to aging, and this means that they often have to spend a lot of their money on medications that are not covered by provincial health-care plans. Shockingly, three out of four women don't have a personal savings account. Single women and women of colour are far more likely to live in poverty than white men. The average income for a Canadian male is still significantly higher than it is for a Canadian woman. Difficulty in paying bills and making ends meet leads to feelings of anxiousness, sleeplessness, guilt, irritability, and persistent physical symptoms. Poverty is stressful and tiring: many women work at two or three jobs in order to survive and cannot afford some of the conveniences that make life easier.

Spending Addictions

Spending addictions can lead to unnecessary poverty or aggravate already "slim pickins." When you consider the stressors of the traditional workplace as well as the stressors discussed in Chapter 4, you can see why it's natural for women to seek out something that makes them feel better about themselves. For millions of North American women, the "feel good" drug they seek out comes in the form of material items: housewares, cosmetics, apparel, shoes, and accessories; these women have developed what's known as a "shopping addiction." The Internet only fuels the shopping frenzies.

For a significant portion of women, gambling is where their money goes; increasing numbers of Canadian women are developing a gambling addiction as more and more casinos open up across the country. Gambling is a spending addiction that provides a sort of euphoria. It is more related to drug addiction than to shopping. Women who shop have a tangible item that makes them feel good, such as a new scarf or shoes. They can hold and feel the item they've purchased—it's something "real" even though it may not be a realistic expenditure. Gambling offers no tangible item other than a return on the investment, which 99.9 percent of the time gets re-gambled. Slot machines are highly addictive because they give credit rather than coins for money and operate at high speed. Women can easily spend hundreds of dollars per day.

Like other addictions, spending addictions provide a high, an escape from the underlying stressors of family life, relationships, or work. They may also be an escape from feeling impoverished. Spending addictions are directly related to women and poverty in that they cause women to incur much more debt than they need to. They ought to be treated as addictions, however, and not simply as a tendency to run up debts.

The "feel good" feeling that women get when they shop can be recreated through bargain hunting. Bargain hunting fulfils the same needs as a shopping-addiction, but costs less. Both involve hunting for an item and feeling great (high) about the purchase. (Many times I wind up calling my shopping purchases the "mistakes in my closet.") Although this is not a serious financial planning tip, women may benefit from adjusting their shopping destinations if shopping is a serious addiction. Instead of going to a "first run" clothing store, they should check out second-hand clothing stores or what I call "Good Wills in Good Neighbourhoods." These can produce even more fantastic highs when you walk away with an item that cost you only $10 instead of $100. Some women become so addicted to bargains it's hard for them to go back to regular stores when the good times return. Just a thought. It worked for me. Of course, Ebay is another story. Be careful!

6 BODIES AND AGING

As women, we can experience a great deal of stress just by thinking about our bodies; put another way, we seldom *stop* thinking about our bodies. Whether it involves an unhealthy fixation on our weight and physical appearance, the need to plan our lives around our menstrual cycles, having to make choices about our fertility, or the normal changes of our reproductive life cycles, our stress is intricately wound around how *we* feel about our bodies and how our bodies make *us* feel. This chapter explores the role body image plays in stress and then discusses hormonal factors that contribute to stress, anxiety, and depression.

Body Image

Most women are stressed by what they see in the mirror. A third of the women in Canada believe they are overweight, even when their body weight is normal for their size, height, and age. Not surprisingly, 90 percent of all eating disorders are diagnosed in women. In Canada, 1 in 9 women aged 14–25 has an eating disorder, but this is certainly an under-reported problem. A *New York Times* poll found that 36 percent of girls aged 13–17 want to change their looks; at least 10 percent of girls 14 and over suffer from an eating disorder.

> We were on a family vacation last summer, and at dinner, my seven-year-old daughter refused to finish her meal because she said she thought she was "fat." I have always struggled with my own weight, and I suddenly began to wonder if she had

been overhearing me in other conversations. I was very upset and simply told her she should never worry about something like that. Now we never talk about weight around her, but she could have gotten that message from hundreds of places. My daughter is so bright, beautiful, and full of promise; now I worry that her innocence over her body and sense of well-being have been lost.

During a recent lecture tour, a man asked me to describe what it feels like to be a woman in our culture. My answer was the following: "We get up in the morning and it begins. Continuous bombardment of beauty and fitness images from all forms of media. The result is that we are never beautiful enough, thin enough, or young enough to feel good about ourselves. Wherever we go, our appearance is watched and judged. Although women may be able to make peace with their appearance and accept their bodies, it is next to impossible for most women to feel truly beautiful." The man was stunned and said, "This can't be true; it sounds so painful to be a woman." I then turned to the rest of the audience and said: "If there's any woman in this room who feels what I just said is inaccurate, please raise your hand." Not one of the roughly 100 women raised her hand. Instead, they quietly nodded to me; some mouthed "It's so true."

Women's bodies are objects in our current culture, used to uphold, and impose, impossible standards of beauty. No woman is immune to this powerful psychological attack. And so ours is a culture in which women see their bodies as objects, too. Experts in women, health, and body image see a literal separation between mind, body, and spirit, sometimes known as mind-body dualism.

A woman's relationship with her body is complex. Her body is her source of power. When the body ages or is otherwise deemed to be less attractive, the woman suffers a loss of power. When a woman relies on her body to empower her, her real autonomy is interfered with—her own power to run her own life. By focusing on our bodies, we have lost many of our strengths as women. Some authors suggest that this is a deliberate ploy by the male-dominated world to distract us from the business of real liberation, which, as Gloria Steinem has said, is a revolution, not public relations.

Because the body size can be manipulated and changed through eating, dieting, starving, exercising, and so on, the body has become a live sculpture for millions of women. Essentially, they sculpt their bodies, using food as the clay in their attempt to achieve the size and shape that is considered ideal. But since food is more than just clay for women—it can be a source of comfort or torture—many women have developed complex and often contradictory behaviour to have their "comfort" and "clay," too. (Of course, facelifts, liposuction, breast augmentation, and other cosmetic surgery—including Botox treatments, which amount to injecting poison into the face to eliminate wrinkles—also serve this "live sculpture" theme. For the purposes of this chapter, I'm limiting the discussion to weight issues.)

If a woman wants to sculpt herself into a thin body, then she has to control how much clay to use, which could mean either severely limiting the food she takes in or purging after eating. If she wants to surround herself with flesh and comfort and make her body large, then she may binge on food without purging. If a woman wants to sculpt herself into a skeleton, which for her would symbolize her self-restraint and control, then she will deny herself comfort at all costs and simply refuse food altogether. She would rather die than show that she wants comfort.

Since much of a woman's self-worth is invested in her outer appearance (whether she admits it or not), feelings of self-loathing and low self-esteem are driven by how she perceives her own body—that is, by her body image. When a woman is depressed, her feelings of low self-esteem cannot be separated from her body image. Matters get even more complicated when we address social issues, such as the aftermath of sexual abuse. When her body has been invaded, a woman often manipulates her body size to make it less appealing to future attackers.

This section looks at the *behaviour* associated with attempts to sculpt various body sizes and the *meaning* of different body sizes. There are just as many women, for example, who have an interest in being large as there are women who have an interest in being thin. This section will not tell you how to get down—or up—to your desired weight, but it will outline some of the reasons *why* you may desire the weight you desire. Once you understand why you want a particular body, it will be clearer to you that your body image and your resulting behaviour are causing you stress.

What It Means to Be Thin

At one point in our culture, to be thin meant to be poor and hungry; a plump woman was a wealthy, successful woman. (Ever seen a Mae West film?) But the emergence of two significant trends changed the perception of "thin." First, food-distribution patterns changed in North America, and nutritious foods became more expensive than low-nutrient, fattening foods. Fat started to be associated with the lower classes. Second, as women began to flood the workplace, the female body became masculinized. The successful woman was a tall, thin, mannish woman who did not show evidence, on her body, of being female or of harbouring reproductive organs. The beauty standard that we see on runways and in magazines reflects the masculinization of the female form. Since women instinctively realize that their bodies must be controlled in order to look masculine, they have come to associate feminine curves with loss of control. The successful woman can look like a man because she *controls* her food intake. Some experts add that control over internal impulses such as hunger is perceived as the conquering of animal instincts. The unsuccessful woman cannot control her food intake and therefore takes on the rounder shape that is rejected by our society. (These stereotypes tend to be limited to white Western society, however; many black women, for example, like being large, and in Caribbean countries, larger women are considered attractive.) Controlling one's food intake is synonymous with self-control, self-discipline, and, ultimately, success—another facet of the power struggle.

For many women, controlling the shape of their body gives them a sense of accomplishment. The irony is that a thin body actually leaves the impression of ineffectiveness, delicateness, and frailty.

Achieving Thinness

For 2 percent of the female population in North America, starving and purging are considered normal ways to control weight. Experts estimate that the number is actually much higher than this, since many women successfully hide their disorder for years. The two most common eating disorders involving starvation are *anorexia nervosa* (not eating) and *bulimia nervosa* (binging followed by purging)—both briefly touched on in Chapter 3. Women will purge after a binging episode by inducing vomiting or abusing laxatives, diuretics, and thyroid hormones. The most horrifying examples occur in women with Type 1 diabetes who deliberately withhold their insulin to control their weight.

As an aside, perhaps the most accepted purging behaviour is *over-exercising*. Today, rigorous, strenuous exercise has become socially acceptable feminine behaviour. A skeleton with biceps is the current ideal, one that is reinforced by several female celebrities.

Eating disorders are diseases of control that primarily affect women, although more men have developed these disorders in recent years. Bulimics and anorexics are usually overachievers in other aspects of their lives; they view excess weight as an announcement to the world that they are going "out of control." This view becomes more distorted as time goes on, until the act of eating food in public (in bulimia) or at all (in anorexia) is perceived to add up to a loss of control.

In anorexia, the person's emotional and sensual desires are channelled through food. These desires are so great that the anorexic fears that once she eats she'll never stop, since her appetite/desire knows no natural boundaries; the fear of food drives the disease. As noted in Chapter 3, many experts believe that eating disorders are addictions and that the "drug" is a sense of control.

Most of us find it easier to relate to the bulimic than the anorexic. Bulimics express their loss of control through binging in the same way that someone else may yell at his or her children. Bulimics then purge to regain their control. There is a feeling of comfort for bulimics in both the binge and the purge. Bulimics are sometimes referred to as "failed anorexics" because they'd starve if they could. Anorexics, however, are masters of control. They never break. I once asked a recovering anorexic the dumb question, "But didn't you get *hungry*?" Her response was that the hunger pangs made her feel powerful. The more intense the hunger, the more powerful she felt; the power actually gave her a high, reinforcing the addiction theory.

The onset of anorexia is traditionally seen during adolescence, when the female body is changing dramatically. Controlling her food intake is viewed by the teenage anorexic as controlling her puberty—trying to stop her body from changing into a woman's. However, this disease is also seen in a number of older women, in their 30s and 40s. Here, the woman may also be expressing her desire to stop her body from changing, but in her case, the change she is trying to stop is the aging process itself. A number of older anorexic women get overlooked and aren't included in the anorexic population because they don't fit the profile (they aren't "young"), even though the evidence of their eating disorder may be more pronounced because of their age.

What It Means to Be Fat

Being fat—and the overeating behaviour that *causes* us to be fat—is perceived by many to be a very public rebellion against the role many women are asked to play in this society. If you are overweight, it's important that you explore what being fat means to *you*, personally, and that includes understanding the issues you have surrounding food addiction.

As women, we are usually the ones who do the purchasing and preparing of food for our families. We are the nurturers and providers. But at the same time, we are continuously being deluged with those impossible standards of beauty, fitness, and thinness through the media. How do these conflicting images affect us? For many women, the effect is a feeling of powerlessness. For many women, manipulating the body size to be bigger by eating food may be a way to express unconscious desires to achieve more control over their lives.

Specialists in compulsive overeating disorders stress that the only way to help women lose weight is to help them understand what conscious or unconscious needs are being met by the fat. Therapists who work with women on weight-loss issues observe that fat both isolates a woman and publicly proclaims her a failure. Women, of course, know this, and sometimes they use it to psychological advantage. In other words, to the woman, the fat can "excuse" her from being successful in two specific arenas: the sexual and the financial (i.e., careers). Many women fear being perceived in a sexual way by male colleagues (they may have had negative experiences when they've been so perceived/noticed in the past).

On the flip side, many women who have never had success in their lives (sexual or financial) use their fat as a way to remain isolated. This allows them to say to themselves: "If I were thin, I'd be successful." The fatness becomes the reason for failed attempts at personal success, shielding women from their own inner demons and fears, keeping them from the successes they really want.

When Fat Means "Mother"

For many women, especially those who gained their weight after childbirth, fat has nothing to do with sexuality or personal/financial success. It has to do with their relationship with their mother and their own feelings about nurturing and being a mother. After all, it is a mother's breasts that initially nurture us, and it is through our mothers that we learn about food and behaviour around food. Our mothers are also the source of love, comfort, emotional support, and our sense of what is acceptable. Even when we do not get this from own mothers, we still associate mothering with these things. Therapists have observed that body size and eating get tangled up in mother-daughter relationships and can have varied meanings for the overweight woman. In other words, your fat can be telling your mother anything from "I'm a big girl and can look after myself" to "I'm a mess and *can't* look after myself." Some daughters use fat to reject their mother's standards or to express anger at their mother for inadequate nurturing. In other cases, the fat represents an unconscious desire to incorporate your mother into your body because she's soothing and nurturing. It's a rather brilliant way of taking your mother with you wherever you go.

When Fat Means "Screw You"

Many women find that their fat expresses anger at the beauty standard and restrictive sexual role they're asked to play. The fat is not "protection" but a deliberate attempt to offend the world. Here, the fat says to the world, "Screw you! If you *really* want to get to know me, then you'll take the time to penetrate my layers. Otherwise, *I* don't want to know you!"

The Act of Getting Fat: Compulsive Eating

When we hear "eating disorder," we usually think about anorexia or bulimia. Many people, however, binge without purging. This is also known as *binge eating disorder* (a.k.a. *compulsive overeating*). In this case, the binging is still an announcement to the world that "I'm out of control." Those who purge their binging behaviour are hiding their lack of control. Those who binge and never purge are *advertising* their lack of control. The purger is passively asking for help; the binger who doesn't purge is aggressively asking for help. It's the same disease with a different result.

There is a controversial further layer when it comes to compulsive overeating, one that's often rejected by the overeater: the *desire* to get fat may be behind the compulsion. Many people who overeat insist that fat is a consequence of eating food, not a *goal*. Many therapists who deal with overeating disagree, believing that if a woman admits that she has an emotional interest in actually being large, she may be closer to stopping her compulsion to eat.

Do You Have a Body-Image Problem?

Few women can say that they like their bodies, while most women distort their body size in their own mind. Our obsession over our bodies becomes a problem requiring therapy or counselling when it interferes with other aspects of our lives. Compulsive weighing, spending a lot of your time worrying about your weight or your body, and practising one of the eating behaviours discussed in this chapter (starving, binging and/or purging, over-exercising) is a sign that you need help, even if you don't exhibit signs of anxiety or depression.

Most women set their desired-weight goal at roughly 10 pounds *under* their ideal weight; many women who think they are overweight are either at an ideal weight or 10 pounds underweight. Normal body fat for a healthy woman is 22–25 percent; most models and actresses have roughly 10 percent body fat. Experts suggest you ask yourself five questions to help establish what a reasonable weight would be for you:

1. What is the lowest weight you have maintained as an adult for at least one year?

2. What is the largest size of clothing you feel you can "look good" in and how much do you need to weigh to wear that size?

3. Think of someone you know (versus a model or actress) who is of your age and height and who appears to be a "normal" weight. What does that person *actually* weigh?

4. What weight can you live with?

5. What does your cultural background value in terms of body size and shape?

Body-Image Quiz

You may have a body-image problem if you

- are preoccupied or obsessed with food and weight;
- narrow your food choices as the days go on (i.e., this week it's no fat; next week it's no carbohydrates, etc.);
- insist you're fat when you're not;
- feel guilty or ashamed to eat in public;
- exercise to lose weight rather than to be fit;
- are overly concerned about your appearance;
- experience mood changes in association with your appearance (i.e., self-loathing after eating or depression or sadness after you've eaten a big meal);
- see only two types of bodies: fat or thin, versus healthy, normal, average, etc.;
- have problems feeling good about yourself after eating;
- avoid public or family gatherings because you don't look good enough;
- don't participate in activities that require you to wear shorts, a bathing suit, etc.; and
- avoid sexual relations because you hate your body.

Fitting Our Bodies into a Man's World

As I've mentioned throughout this book, our society, our buildings, and our entire economy were designed for a male body, not a woman's. The "office bathroom" story in Chapter 1 is an obviously alarming example of the stress that can surround a normal function. In this section, we will see how normal female functions can be the source of a great deal of stress when we are not allowed, literally, to be ourselves.

Premenstrual Discomforts

Virtually all women in their childbearing years have premenstrual discomforts. As we age, our premenstrual signs can become more severe, especially as we approach our perimenopause, a term that means "around menopause," which is usually somewhere in our mid-to-late 40s. Premenstrual signs occur roughly 14 days before your period and disappear when you get your period or just after. Traditionally, women's complaints about premenstrual signs have either been viewed as psychological or been written off as part of the biological lot of women. Many women have difficulty admitting they suffer from these symptoms for fear of compromising their position in the workplace, but virtually all women experience some premenstrual signs. It's how *you* experience these signs and how severely they affect *you* that determines how much stress you endure. Also, a woman's premenstrual discomforts can worsen when she's under stress (I discuss this in Chapter 1).

Ninety percent of women who menstruate experience premenstrual signs of some sort. Of these women, about 50 percent will experience the more traditional premenstrual signs, such as breast tenderness, bloating, food cravings, irritability, and mood swings. These signs, for many women, are often perceived as an indication that their bodies are "in tune" or "on schedule" and that all is well. In other words, premenstrual signs are natural markers of a healthy menstrual cycle. If you fall into this first group, you may find that by moderately adjusting your diet or adding one or two of the dietary or herbal supplements that will be discussed in Part 3, you can dramatically reduce your premenstrual discomfort.

From 35 to 40 percent of menstruating women experience the same signs as the first group, but in a more severe form. In other words, they have *really* tender breasts, so sensitive that they hurt if someone just lightly touches them; they suffer severe bloating, to the extent that they gain about five pounds before their period; instead of having just food cravings, they may suddenly have voracious appetites; they may find that they've gone beyond feeling merely irritable and have become impossible to be around; and so on. Even these more severe signs are considered to be normal. If you fall into this group, you may find that more rigorous dietary adjustments and supplements, in combination with herbal remedies and physical activity, can significantly lessen your discomfort. You may also benefit from ruling out other causes of your discomforts and may even want to explore natural progesterone supplements.

Roughly 3–10 percent of menstruating women (the latest statistics hover around 3–4 percent) suffer from incapacitating discomforts that affect their ability to function and interfere with their quality of life. They experience, among other things, profound mood swings; sudden, unexplainable sadness; irritability; sudden or unexplainable anger; feelings of anxiety or of being on edge; depression; hopelessness; self-deprecating thoughts, and the gamut of physical discomforts (tender breasts, bloating, and so on). In the psychiatric literature, even women with hysterectomies and oophorectomies (removal of their ovaries) are found to experience these symptoms. It is considered sound practice, and good medicine, to offer this group of women antidepressants as a treatment for premenstrual syndrome (PMS), even though incapacitating discomforts can still be managed through natural remedies. If you fall into this group, it's important to first rule out other causes of your physical and emotional discomforts, such as other stress aggravators or an underlying depression that has social causes and is a response to the conditions of your life (see Chapter 2). If you're taking synthetic hormones or medications, it's possible that your reactions to these (if you have any) are being aggravated by your own fluctuating hormones around the time of your period. Next, take a long hard look at your diet and activity patterns. Adjusting your diet, adding supplements and herbs, and becoming more active can really make a difference. Finally, you may benefit from natural progesterone supplements, and you should discuss this treatment with your doctor. I urge you to consider synthetic hormones, antidepressants, anti-anxiety agents, and other medications *only* as a very last resort. These are strong medications that carry a long list of side-effects. For more information, consult my book *Managing PMS Naturally*.

Pregnancy

Today, the stress involved with pregnancy is not just around the physical discomforts (there are dozens of normal discomforts of pregnancy listed by trimester in most pregnancy books) or the hormonal shifts that occur in pregnancy. There now seems to be much more to consider. The moment a woman announces her pregnancy, she has all kinds of decisions to make. She has to struggle with moral decisions about prenatal tests, not an easy thing given all the "probabilities and outcomes" that surround such tests. She must also decide what kinds of practitioner she wants (doula, midwife, obstetrician, etc.) and whether to birth at home, in hospital, and so on. Then there are the stresses involved when the pregnancy does not go as planned: women can develop high-risk pregnancies and many different health problems, such as diabetes. Or, the woman may lose her baby; one in six pregnancies ends in miscarriage and that number climbs as women age. Factor into all of this the double shift—having to work and manage a family—and that spells STRESS in capital letters.

Motherhood

Major stress often begins with motherhood—when the baby is brought home. Sources of stress include the isolation many women experience during the postpartum adjustment period, as well as problems surrounding breastfeeding. Review Chapter 4 for more details.

Gynecological Problems

Consider how all of the following garden-variety gynecological problems (listed alphabetically) can add to, or create, stress in your life:

- Bleeding between periods
- Endometriosis
- Fibroids
- Heavy bleeding or "flooding" due to perimenopause
- Infections and inflammation (such as yeast, vaginitis, or vulvitis)
- Missed periods (when women are stressed about being pregnant, the stress can delay the period even longer)
- Pelvic inflammatory disease (PID)
- Side-effects from taking the Pill
- Sexually transmitted diseases (e.g., herpes, chlamydia, HIV, hepatitis)
- Vaginal dryness or itching

We're not going to "go there" in this book, but you can consult *The Gynecological Sourcebook* for more information. Just being aware of the many things women deal with below-the-belt, all the time, is enough to stress you out!

Aging and Menopause

When the first signs of menopause started to interfere with my life, I was angry. I had done my research and was prepared to age naturally and gracefully. My one resolve was: no hormones. I have a job that involves a lot of travelling in very rough conditions. When working out in the field a couple of years ago, I got my first "gushy," almost-period "flood." It was early, and I was not prepared. When you're 49 years old and have to stuff leaves inside your undies and rip up your clothing to manufacture creative tampons, it's time to re-evaluate your thinking about HRT. I was the only woman on this trip; I didn't want to give up a project that I'd worked so hard to fund just because of "woman stuff" that was beyond my control. In fact, I was respected by the men on the trip; my being a woman wasn't a problem for them—but it sure as hell was a problem for me that week.

As women extend their childbearing years more dramatically than ever, many find themselves at a crossroads when they approach menopause, or the banner birthday: 50. Many women at this age have just had a child or have a toddler at home. Books on menopause still cover issues such as "empty nest syndrome" even though so many of today's women are still building the nest. Or, worse, they're trying to get adult children to leave the nest. Studies show that women whose children won't leave experience far more stress than women whose children have finally "flown the nest." Changes in the job market have necessitated that young adults stay longer in school, and thus many of them can't afford to leave home until they're close to 30.

As they approach 50, women may find themselves caring for their 70- or 80-something parents as well as their children, which is why the label "the sandwich generation" is so often used. The stress of caring for small children, teens, or young adult children who haven't left home is often combined with the stress of caring for aging parents who may be developing, among a host of other chronic ailments, Alzheimer's disease. As women cross the threshold from parent to caregiver, they will be faced with the hard facts of aging: they'll need to negotiate care for aging parents in an age when our elderly are being warehoused. There are not enough facilities for the numbers of old people who need them, nor are the facilities that are in place well staffed. In a U.S. study, one-quarter of the women surveyed were caring for an aging parent either in their own home or in a facility.

Women who are widowed, divorced, or separated at this point in their lives often experience anxiety about their own economic future. And for many, having no life partner is the source of fears of loneliness and stress over aging alone.

As all of these social factors converge, there are also real concerns over the physical health problems that increase with age. Women worry about their hearts, breasts, bones, and hormones, all of which are the objects of debate and discussion among medical experts. Considering that many women are just beginning to *really* live when they reach menopause, a good proportion of them feel like shouting: "Somebody tell them to turn back the clock! I'm just gettin' rollin'!"

Clearly, our attitudes about aging are shifting dramatically. In 2001 over a million women were reported to be between the ages of 50 and 54 in Canada alone, while almost 20 million women in the U.S. were between 45 and 54—the largest number of women in that age group in U.S. history.

One of the most stressful things about aging is agism, discrimination against people on the basis of their age. One woman who recently turned 60 told me that she began to realize within the last year or so that she could not "get service" the way she used to. Male servers in restaurants ignored her; male retailers ignored her when she was in a store. She used the term "non-person" to describe how turning 60 made her feel.

When we experience our age, or a physical vulnerability, in this way, our life takes on a new meaning and we begin to look at it differently. Gail Sheehy, author of *Passages*, refers to this as a "task of reflection." Upon reflection like this (did we "live well?," are we happy?, were we good people?, are there things we still want or need to do?, etc.), we might experience stress, but it can be a good stress in that it allows us to live with more passion and feeling, and to cross into another stage of life. At this new stage, our health, for example, suddenly becomes very important to us; many people become physically active for the first time or dramatically change their lifestyle habits—eating well, quitting smoking, and so on.

Just to give you an idea of how much longer we're living, in 1994 about 33 million North Americans were over 65. Today, over 100 million North Americans are over 65. And by the year 2010, there will be three times that figure.

Coping with Menopause

Native American folklore records that we are in the midst of massive earth changes that will climax around 2013. It's been said that these earth changes will bring heat, floods, and incredible upheaval to the world's population. By then, over 50 million women will have achieved menopause and will have gone through their own heat (via hot flashes), floods (via heavy bleeding), and upheaval. Some question whether we are entering a "mass" or "collective" menopause. Earth changes notwithstanding, the mass menopause that will take place in the next few years will be felt. Your menopause, in many ways, is a social menopause—a time for our culture to stop and change the way we think about aging.

But there are, of course, some physical and emotional consequences of menopause: as estrogen begins to dwindle, women will experience physical symptoms such as erratic periods, hot flashes, and vaginal dryness. There isn't solid evidence suggesting that estrogen loss leads to irritability, mood swings, melancholy, and so on, but since estrogen functions as a weak antidepressant, it's not surprising that moods may swing as estrogen decreases. Some experts believe that emotional symptoms during menopause are actually caused by a rise in the follicle stimulating hormone (FSH), the hormone that signals the ovaries to "spit out" the follicle, which refers to the egg in the early stage of the cycle. As the menstrual cycle changes and the ovaries' egg supply dwindles, FSH is secreted in very high amounts and reaches a lifetime peak—as much as 15 times higher than in women of childbearing age—in an effort to move the remaining eggs; it's the body's way of trying to jump-start the ovarian engine.

Ironically, the only other time in a woman's life when her FSH levels are as high as they are in menopause is during her puberty. (This may be why the classic mother/daughter "hormone clash" tends to occur when a daughter is entering puberty and the mother is entering menopause. At this stage, both mother and daughter are more sex-hormone matched, in terms of hormonal levels, than at other times in their relationship.) In fact, the erratic up-and-down moods of puberty mirror the mood swings that can characterize menopause, and they may both be accentuated by the presence of higher levels of FSH.

Every woman entering menopause will experience a change in her menstrual cycle. However, not all women will experience hot flashes or even notice vaginal changes. This is particularly true if a woman is overweight. And, of course, many women go through menopause without experiencing changes in their moods. It is an absolute myth to assume that mood swings always accompany menopause or that women who suffer from premenstrual symptoms will always experience more severe menopausal symptoms than other women.

Most mental health experts agree that the blues that women experience during menopausal years are rooted in the psychological fear of aging and the stress associated with the physical symptoms (hot flashes and so on) of menopause. If you're taking hormone replacement therapy (HRT) because you think it will cure any serious depression you're experiencing, you're mistaken. Hormone therapy will relieve your night sweats and any resulting insomnia, as well as anxiety related to your menopausal symptoms, and since you'll be better rested and calmer, you'll be able to cope with daily stress more effectively and positively; but if you are depressed to the extent where you can't function normally, you need to seek out counselling, treatment, or support groups with other women who have experienced menopause.

Age before Beauty

Although space does not allow me to elaborate too much, I want to emphasize how dramatic the stress of aging is. Aging compels many women, for example, to contemplate medical procedures that may prove dangerous, ranging from a host of cosmetic surgeries to Botox injections. The latter treatment involves the injection of small amounts of a toxin into a woman's face; possible side-effects include partial facial paralysis. What's worse, even though Botox is clearly a dramatic, if not outrageous, "treatment" for aging, it is not openly questioned or debated by the medical community.

7

DIVORCE AND LOSS

Statistics Canada predicts that by 2016 the number of families run by single mothers will have climbed to roughly 1.6 million, up from today's 1 million. The vast majority—80 percent—of single mothers are "single" as a result of divorce. And that doesn't account for the number of single women who have ended common-law relationships. Whether relationships end on good terms or bad, the feelings of loss can account for tremendous stress.

Then there is loss of a spouse or partner through death. We are currently seeing an enormous number of younger widows, in their 30s and 40s, because of higher rates of cancers, car accidents, and drug abuse in the young adult population. Grief is a significant cause of stress and poor health.

The deaths of other family members greatly contribute to stress, too. Women routinely cope with the loss of parents, siblings, and friends, and are particularly stricken with grief when they have lost a child. This chapter explores the emotional impact of loss through divorce, a failed relationship, and death.

Divorce

Many books and websites offer practical advice on the highly complex subject of divorce. For the purposes of this book, divorce will be explored in the context of stress. Divorced women are very vulnerable to stress, and they experience higher than average rates of anxiety and depression, alcoholism, and suicide. Even though women may be happier emotionally without their spouse, they still must deal with the stress coming from financial matters, such as income and child support, as well as safety matters, if they left an abusive partner. Women are also subjected to a decline in their social status. They are suddenly viewed as a single woman and are often not invited to couples' events or dinner parties. They may also be stigmatized by certain family members and cultural groups.

Divorce stress is on the rise because divorces are on the rise. In 1987, when the Divorce Act in Canada allowed marriages to end after one year of separation instead of three, the divorce rate peaked. The year 1998 for some reason saw a 2 percent climb in the divorce rate, too.

Women find it easier emotionally to leave an unhappy marriage or relationship than to be left. When a woman is left by her partner, especially when the abandonment is a surprise (for example, her partner admits to an affair or offers no explanation at all), the breakup feels like a death, and a long period of grieving may ensue.

Divorces are almost always intensified when lawyers are involved—often unnecessarily. Lawyers tend to create rather than resolve conflict, especially when they tell you to be on the lookout for all kinds of negative behaviour from your ex, which is their job.

> When I left my husband, we had just our house, which was heavily mortgaged, simple belongings, and separate credit cards and bank accounts. We had no children. It seemed reasonable to just split everything up ourselves, but people kept saying to me, "See a lawyer before you do anything." When I finally consulted a lawyer, she suggested we do up an agreement and told me to ask my husband about his pension and RRSPs because I'm entitled to half of that. I didn't want to do that, but I approached the subject with my husband nonetheless. He was furious; he felt that I was being sneaky by having gone to a lawyer, that this was a sign that I didn't trust him. He had not seen one and had no intention of doing so. He felt that he was experiencing a loss of income due to our parting (I made more money than he did) and didn't understand why his pension and modest RRSPs had to be dragged into it. Then the lawyer started being a devil in my ear, telling me that "people may say one thing, but later when they're angry, do another. Get it in writing." It all sounded perfectly reasonable, but my husband was in so much pain and it was so difficult to broach these subjects, I just stopped dealing with the lawyer. We sold our house, split the profits, and I selected the items from the house I wanted. It wasn't seamless, and I might do things differently today, but I think it would have been a lot worse had we involved lawyers. I have no regrets. We live separately without a legal divorce. The deal is that if ever one of us decides to remarry, we'll get a legal divorce then. We

would have spent more money paying for the divorce than anything that might have come out of it.

Women can be emotionally fragile during a divorce, particularly if they are grieving, and many of them make the mistake of giving all the decision-making powers to their lawyer. This leaves them feeling even more powerless. Conflicts may escalate without the woman's knowledge if something she said is retold out of context, causing the divorcing partner to feel betrayed or to become more aggressive.

In *Kramer vs. Kramer,* one of the first films to truly capture the pain and no win situation of divorce, Meryl Streep plays Joanna, a depressed housewife who leaves Ted, played by Dustin Hoffman, who is left to parent their little boy. In a bitter custody battle, Joanna's lawyer accuses Ted of negligence because the child had fallen down in his care and hurt himself. Joanna had merely told her lawyer that the child had had a fall and had hurt himself; she hadn't intended to accuse her ex-husband. It is her lawyer who uses the boy's accident as a sign of Ted's incompetence. Ted feels betrayed and even less willing to negotiate; Joanna feels betrayed by her own lawyer, since he distorted a candid remark of hers and used it in court. This film also represents another truth about divorce: more women than men tend to leave their relationship these days. Often a "psychological divorcing" of the spouse has taken place long before the actual leaving. But when women leave, many of the male partners become aggressive in the ensuing legal battle.

Unfortunately, lawyers are a necessary evil—especially when custody and child support are involved. More than half of all child-support payments go unpaid, while a woman's standard of living falls anywhere from 27–45 percent in the first year after a divorce. A man's income typically rises by 10 percent. Women are often left with terrible settlements because the men outspend them in a divorce. The opposite is true as well.

As has already been noted, divorce stress stems from both the emotional issues involved with leaving or being left and the financial mess that needs to be sorted out. Moving and relocating—which often accompany a divorce—are considered stressful enough in the best of times. Divorce can be a stress pressure cooker that explodes.

When you're going through a divorce, the services of a mediator instead of a lawyer often reduces the stress. The fair division of uncomplicated assets can be negotiated through a mediator. Divorces become more complicated when children are involved. Mediation can often help to establish fair co-parenting arrangements, but most of the problems with children and divorce revolve around negotiating fair financial support and access, the domain of lawyers.

Most of the advice on divorce that you'll find on the Internet and in books focuses on financial and legal issues. Frequently missing is information on the grieving process. Divorce, or the loss of any relationship, can be as painful as the death of a loved one. Reducing the stress of divorce starts with understanding that you are going through a loss, not just a "divorce" or a "breakup." Loss and grief are also enormous energy drains.

Loss

Out of the roughly 13 million widowed North Americans, more than 11 million are women. Women over 55 represent nearly 65 percent of the widowed population. Widows represent nearly 50 percent of the 20 million women in the U.S. who are 65 and older; of those, less than 10 percent remarry. Ten to 20 percent suffer long-term health problems such as prescription drug abuse, depression, alcoholism, and suppressed immunity. Beyond the loss of a spouse, the experience of losing a parent, a sibling, or, most traumatic, a child can propel us into long bouts of grief. The average grieving period is two to five years; it can take that long to adjust to a loss.

It's worth noting that the loss of a pet, for many women, can be met with profound feelings of grief. Perhaps because of embarrassment over the feelings we have for our pets, many of us are afraid to admit to, or express, our grief over a pet's death. For many women, pets are real companions who offer unconditional acceptance and love. They may serve as vessels for many emotions that never get "released" into relationships with our own species. Furthermore, our feelings of guilt over putting our pets to sleep adds another dimension to our grief.

The biggest problem women face when they've suffered a loss is their tendency to deny themselves the time to express their grief. Grief is a necessary adjustment period that cannot be sped up, although it can be delayed. Many women feel compelled to get on with life even though they may not have properly grieved. Holding in grief can be extremely stressful. Experts on loss, such as clergy and mental health professionals, point out that grieving will occur sooner or later; it is a necessary stage of loss that all of us have to go through. There is a distinction between bereavement and grief: grief is a process of feeling and accepting loss; bereavement is the event of loss. You can be bereaved by any loss, not just death: loss of a relationship, job, friends who've moved away; your health, your youth; and even your faith. And you can go through periods of grieving for any of those losses. In short, you are a bereaved person because of a loss; the feelings you have as a result are connected to your grief. The loss of a relationship, person, or other important part of your life is connected to a series of other losses—loss of dreams, hope, financial security, identity, social circle, intimacy, future, best friend, faith, and so on.

What to Expect When You're Grieving

The first thing to remember about grieving is that it is something that can't be denied or avoided. It is a crucial adjustment and transition period. Some authors on grief refer to it as the process by which we seek to find new meaning: we have lost an important point of reference that has defined our lives and we now need to find a new one. People often feel adrift during the grieving period, unable to make decisions and unsure of what they want and of what they're feeling. Some people begin grieving before the loss because they are anticipating it. This is known as anticipatory grief. In many cases, however, anticipatory grief is masked by false hope, especially when we deny that a person is dying or a relationship is ending. Or the opposite occurs: we didn't anticipate feeling as much grief as we do feel. This is common when family members with whom we've had stormy relationships die. We thought we would feel relief, and we are shocked by how much grief we feel.

Depending upon the circumstances of the loss, the following feelings are all common during grieving: sadness, pain, loneliness, frustration, anger, uselessness, helplessness, separation, panic, fog, guilt, disappointment, shock, confusion, depression (characterized by numbness, indifference, and a lack of engagement with your life), emptiness, sense of meaninglessness, fear, feeling alone and unloved, and even relief (common when the loved one died a long, painful death). Physical manifestations of many of these feelings are crying, sleeplessness, change in appetite (some people cannot eat, while others comfort themselves with food), and panic attacks.

Working through Grief

Grief is something that you have to work through at your own pace. Here are the four "tasks" involved in grieving:

Accept the Reality of the Loss.

Many people deny that the loss is real; this is especially true when a relationship is over but the person is still alive and well. When coping with a death, we may have the sense that the person will somehow return, that they are away on a trip; feelings like this often lead to "shrine" behaviour. In the film *Ordinary People,* a bereaved mother, Beth (played by Mary Tyler Moore), goes to such lengths to suppress her grief that she alienates the rest of her family. Buck, her first and favourite son, died in a boating accident. Two years later, his room is exactly as it was, with all of his awards, clothes, and personal items completely intact—as though he would be coming home any day. Beth goes into the room, sits on the bed, and finds comfort, although it is an unhealthy comfort because she is really comforted by "pretending" he isn't dead.

Experience the Pain of Grief.

Don't be afraid to feel your feelings. "You have to feel before you heal" is a trite phrase often used by therapists, but it is a true one, especially with grief. If you delay your natural feelings by trying to deny them, they can come back to haunt you later on. In the same film mentioned above, *Ordinary People*, the surviving sibling (played by Timothy Hutton) tries very hard to repress the pain of grief, but finally feels it so intensely, he cannot deal with it alone. He calls his therapist (played by Judd Hirsh) to help him through the maze of overwhelming emotions. By working through this maze, Hutton discovers that he has been feeling guilty because he was the one who survived and also because he felt responsible for the death of his brother (they were in the same boating accident). His therapist asks him: "What was it that you did that was so terrible?" Hutton answers: "I survived; I hung on to the boat—I stayed with the boat." It is at this point that Hutton, whose bottled-up grief, anger, and guilt had led to a suicide attempt, finally cries for the first time since his brother's death. He realizes that now he can begin the recovery process.

Adjust to Your New Environment.

Your life is different without the person or thing you're grieving over. Do something that acknowledges your new reality, such as joining a bereavement group, disposing of belongings connected with the loss, redecorating your home, drawing up a new will, or planning an activity alone.

Emotionally Relocate Your Lost One.

If your mind were a house, what room would your lost one belong in now that he, she, or "it" is gone? In other words, by relocating the lost person in another place, you are not forgetting about him or her, but you are moving other things, things that are alive and real, into the "living room" or "bedroom."

Grief can take a long time, but as noted above, most people find they are able to work through it and find new meaning to their lives within two to five years. In some cases, grief may be worked through within a few months to a year, but this is not a realistic statistic. Too often, grief can trigger depression, which can last many months.

Factors that will affect the grieving period include the nature of your relationship with the lost one, how prepared you were for the loss, and your own personal history with loss. Unresolved grief from past losses can add up and intensify a fresh one. Other factors influencing your grieving period include whether you have a supportive network of family and friends, your overall mental and emotional health, your spiritual beliefs and touchstones, and other stresses in your life. The cause of a death can also influence grieving, especially if it is stigmatizing, such as death from suicide or murder. Also, grieving can be more difficult if the lost one was someone who was not socially accepted by your family or peers. The funeral rites are another factor. Did you properly say goodbye? People who have lost family members in plane crashes are unable to give their loved ones proper burials when the bodies cannot be recovered. The memorial services in cases such as these are attempts to replace the traditional funeral, but they don't always feel like proper burials.

Depression and Grief

Jessica Lange, in the film *Men Don't Leave*, gives a faithful portrayal of a woman going through a depression brought on by grief. Lange plays a homemaker who lacks marketable skills but must suddenly provide for her two sons after her husband is killed in a car accident. At first, she goes through the normal stages of grieving and seems to be able to make significant changes in her life in response to new financial pressures and realities. She sells her house in a rural area and moves to an apartment in the nearby urban centre. She finds a job with a catering company. She *seems* to be doing great, all things considered. But her life starts to fall apart when loneliness sets in and the stresses of being a single parent become overwhelming. She drifts into a major depression, taking to her bed for five consecutive days. In a particularly poignant scene, one of her sons tries to wake her up, asking her if she's still "tired." Barely able to respond, Lange asks her son if he's hungry. When he replies, "Yes," she drags herself out of bed into a dirty, unkempt kitchen, makes him a peanut butter sandwich, serving it on a paper towel, and gives him tap water to drink when she discovers there is no milk or juice in the house. The kitchen table is piled high with dirty laundry and dishes. The child sits at a clean corner of the table, quietly eating his sandwich, while his mother heads back to bed. She awakens the next day out of what looks like a fitful sleep, stumbles into the kitchen to feed herself—cold spaghetti out of a can. What's so accurate about this portrayal is that the depression doesn't immediately follow the death of the husband; it takes several months to manifest. But it is still triggered by feelings of loss and grief.

Mental health experts say that if profound feelings of sadness and an inability to eat, sleep, or concentrate persist beyond three months, your grief may have developed into a full-blown depression. However, since the grieving process can take a long time, it is perhaps more accurate to say that depression is sometimes a necessary part of the grieving process. When we are forced to let go of an old way of being or thinking, depression may be the state that many of us enter in order to deal with the crisis and hopefully "emerge" more true to ourselves. Whether depression entails a slowing down or a complete halt, its symptoms may be necessary if we're to successfully do an emotional "triptik" of re-routing and changing direction, so we can either continue along the road to self-actualization or perhaps discover it for the first time.

Certain people are more likely to become depressed after a loss than others. People with a history of depression, people who have lost a relationship of many years, and people who have lost a relationship that was unresolved (losses such as the latter lead to profound feelings of guilt and regret) are more likely to suffer from depression.

When to Seek Help with Your Grief

There is a normal period of grieving that can't be denied (two to five years), but there is also grief that persists beyond the normal grieving period. Here are some warning signs that indicate you should seek help with a professional grief counsellor:

- Many years have passed, but your grief feels very fresh and intense.
- The death of someone you don't know very well has triggered fresh feelings of intense grief.
- You dwell on the death or loss of your loved one in conversations with friends, to the point where they tell you that you need help.
- You have not disposed of the personal effects of your loved one, even though the normal grieving period has passed.
- You are going through a long bout of depression.
- You like to wear the clothing of the lost one long after she or he is gone.
- You feel suicidal.
- You are worried you will die from the same cause as your lost one.
- You begin to idolize your lost one.
- You're abusing drugs, alcohol, or food (you may be eating compulsively).
- You've isolated yourself and will not go out.

If you are grieving over a relationship loss, the following signs indicate that you should seek help:

- You are obsessing over the relationship and can't think about anything else.
- You want revenge. You're consumed with trying to get even with your ex-partner to the point where you may escalate or initiate an unnecessary legal battle.
- You've worn out your friends and family by constantly talking about your circumstances and/or refusing to take advice when it is given.

Signs That Grief Is Passing

Grief counsellors refer to the healing process as a complex period during which various parts of ourselves begin to heal, some more quickly than others. The parts of ourselves involved in the process are the following:

- The relational self, which has to do with the self that relates to other people
- The emotional self, which has to do with the self that feels and is able to express feelings
- The spiritual self, the self that may be finding new faith or coping with lost faith
- The physical self—your physical health

The signs that you are healing vary with the parts of yourself that are beginning to recover. You will know that your relational self is healing when you start to go out with people rather than isolate yourself. Your emotional self is healing when you begin to express your feelings again (crying when you feel like it, for example, instead of bottling up your emotions) and talk to close friends about your feelings instead of saying, "I'm fine." Your spiritual self is healing when you either reconnect with your spiritual community (by going to your usual place of worship), question your faith (or lack of it) and do some reading and critical thinking about old belief systems that may not work for you anymore, or find faith when you were previously not spiritual at all. Your physical self is healing when you are eating well, getting rest, and staying physically active.

Friends in Need

Over the years, many women have confided to me that it is their relationships with other women that get them through hard times. For some women, their best girlfriends are their own family members, such as mothers, daughters, sisters, cousins, aunts, and so on. Most women, however, have at least two or three close female friends who are like their family—friends who have been accepting of them in good times and bad. The real distinction between friends and family members is that a friend is someone with whom we've voluntarily established a relationship, one based on an unspoken rule: reciprocity. This means that there is giving and taking between friends both directly and indirectly, over prolonged periods of time. There is also a mutual assumption that the reciprocity will be maintained indefinitely. Women become friends with people they feel connected to on some level; it could be a common history or shared philosophy of life.

Friends support each other and offer a break from the demands of life. Most studies on women's friendships cited conversation, rather than an activity shared by both friends, as the most valuable element of the friendship. Companionship in the form of talking is really what most women need. The activities surrounding the friendship are just venues in which conversation can take place. Companionship in the form of showing up in times of need is also highly valued, as is companionship in the form of supporting an activity. Women may take courses together, go jogging together, and so on. Their companionship, in this case, is a support system for the activity.

In times of loss, female friends comprise the support networks for the grieving woman. They help her dispose of belongings; wait with her while her ex removes his things from her apartment; goes with her to the funeral home and helps her make the arrangements; helps her remove belongings from her deceased parent's condo; watches her kids while she runs to hospitals. And so on.

But since friendships are voluntary relationships, there are boundaries that many do not cross. Few friends expect of one another financial support, unconditional child care, or accommodation. Friendships can become strained when these boundaries are abused.

> A friend of mine left her boyfriend of nine years and needed a place to stay "for a week." She wound up staying on my couch for over a month, and I finally told her that she needed to find other accommodations and gave her a deadline. She probably would have done the same for me, but I'm not sure I would have allowed myself to overstay like that. She did help with the housework and was conscientious, but she was unemployed and couldn't really contribute financially. When the deadline came for her to go elsewhere, I was angry when she went to another friend's place and was there for about a month, too. People start to feel used after a point. We've all been down and out, but people need to know other people's limits.

Finding Out Who Your Friends Are

A close friend's husband committed suicide at 40, and I was arranging the food for the "shiva"—the Jewish custom of friends visiting the bereaved for the first seven days after a death. I was expecting a pretty large crowd of people. My friend had a small immediate family who were at the house, and friends of some of the family came. But out of all the friends in our circle, I was the only one who was there. None of the others came. I made the terrible mistake of calling people and asking where they were, and people kept saying, "I wanted to give her some time alone," or "Well … I really didn't know him all that well." I was at a loss to explain their behaviour, but my girlfriend told me that she wasn't surprised: "People can't handle it. It's their problem, not mine." In the end, the people who did not come to the shiva did not even send a card or flowers. They simply vanished. I was appalled.

Loss can bring out your friends' true colours. When you experience a loss, some friends may stop calling you. Divorced and widowed women frequently lose friends they made when they were one half of a couple. Suddenly, they're not invited to the same social functions or they notice that people tend to avoid them. Alternatively, someone you may have lost touch with may become surprisingly supportive when you experience a loss.

Sometimes the friends you thought you could count on—they've come through for you in the past—just aren't truly there for you; these friends may be going through rough time themselves, and their lack of support may have nothing to do with their reliability and everything to do with bad timing.

As noted above, friendships have boundaries that don't typically include the provision of financial support, child care, and accommodation. In times of loss, unfortunately, financial problems are frequently part of the loss package. Friendship boundaries can be crossed when too many inquiries are made and unwanted financial advice is dispensed. The other way around can also be a problem: women report that they are often sorry they have disclosed their financial circumstances to friends, as the information can be compromising to the friendship. Generally, friends who lend money to one another or provide each other with free accommodation have long-established histories and an implicit understanding that the act of generosity could not be obtained through any other source.

PART three

MANAGING STRESS

*You know the signs, symptoms,
and chief causes of stress.
This section explores some ways you can reduce stress.*

8 DOWNSHIFTING

Downshifting is a term that emerged in the early 1990s meaning, fittingly, "slowing down." In order to downshift, the first step is to recognize the *need* to do so. Downshifting applies to all aspects of your life: work, relationships, lifestyle, and activities. This chapter shows you some practical ways you can slow down your life and significantly reduce your stress.

Slowing Down Your Work Life

One of the first things to downshift is your job. The best way to do this is to look at whether you even enjoy what you do. If you don't, shouldn't you at least *try t*o do what you love? If you do what you love, you'll love what you do. And you'll feel so much better, even though you may not make as much money.

Why You Should Love Your Work

I had a secure job as a marketing coordinator in an insurance company, but what I really wanted to do was to sell my knit designs. The job wasn't stressful per se, but it was very boring, which caused me a lot of stress because I kept feeling like I was wasting my life. I also had to commute to work an hour each way. One day I dropped into this knitting store not far from me and asked them if they needed any full-time help. The job paid minimum wage, but I could get a 50 percent discount on anything in the store, and the owner didn't mind at all if I brought my knitting into the store and worked on it when we were slow. (She said it would be inspiring for customers.) I returned my leased car, cutting my fixed monthly expenses in half, quit my job, and started to work as a clerk in the knitting store. Soon we started to showcase my knits in the windows, which brought me direct customers. I started to have knitting parties to sell my knits and used the store to advertise the events; I also gave knitting lessons. I wound up leaving a $41,000 job to work for minimum wage, where I earned about $15,000 per year. But the next year, I was earning more than $50,000 because of my knit sales. I really love my life now and am only sorry I didn't pursue my knitting earlier.

Surveys and studies show across the board that stress is created by going to a job you hate every day. "Doing what you love" doesn't mean throwing in the towel and moving to France so you can paint for the rest of your life. It means exploring what you're good at, and/or enjoy doing, to see if there's a way you can earn an income from it. Are there adult courses you could take which would allow you entry into a field you prefer, for example? The promise of a future with the right credentials often reduces chronic stress, since chronic stress springs from the ongoing prospect of "same old/same old." So, although expanding your education or training may involve some short-term stress because of added responsibilities, it will reduce your long-term stress because it will give you a more hopeful future.

Sometimes doing what you love means recognizing that you're not very good at management and would prefer a non-managerial position. Working "in the store" instead of running it is often the solution, one that might even be arranged in the company where you work. On the flip side, sometimes doing what you love means recognizing that you *are* a leader and that your stress is due to your subordinate position. In this case, running your own company, where you have control, would be less stressful, even though it would involve far more responsibility. This explains why home-based businesses are exploding in popularity and why women are starting their own businesses in droves. It's become much easier (particularly for women) to start a home-based business because new technologies allow you to access the global market instantly through the Internet. Moving to a position in a large company that allows you to be an "intrepreneur" is a very satisfying solution when you crave control or want to exercise more leadership. You might want to join the ranks of the millions of "travelling salespeople" who are supplied with gas allowance and work mostly on commission with a small base salary. For many, these positions offer the flexibility and control that enable them to feel autonomous.

Some people downshift by moving to a simple "side-job" with flexible hours that allow them time for their art or main interest. Couriers, postal workers, restaurant servers, and so forth frequently have artistic lifestyles. When the job simply supports their art and doesn't consume their lives, the job is far less stressful because its importance is diminished. Lose one side-job and it's easy to get another; in other words, side-jobs involve *detachment*, while career-jobs involve attachment and far more emotional investment.

Sometimes doing what you love means facing up to the fact that your dream job or profession has become a living nightmare. This is not an easy thing to admit, but it's the point at which, for example, the overworked medical resident in a busy university teaching hospital decides that she's going to head for an under-serviced rural area and become a country doctor. So she won't become the brilliant heart surgeon her family dreamed of; so she won't earn $350,000 per year, not including the conference perks. Instead, she'll settle for a third of that salary in a rural setting where the housing is affordable and people say hello to you.

Pursuing what you love involves these steps:

- Ask yourself if you're happy with your choice of job or career. Being happy is not the same thing as feeling "stable" or "not miserable." It isn't healthy to continue to work in a state of unhappiness.

- Make a list of dream jobs or careers—no matter how silly you think you're being. Did you always want to be a dancer but you're making a living in marketing? Maybe you could pursue administrative or marketing jobs with a dance company or dance theatre. Maybe you could write about dance or start a children's dance school. Have you always wanted to be a farmer? Why not? Organic farming is booming! Dream jobs can also mean parenting! If being a stay-at-home parent is your dream, it's worth pursuing, too.

- Assess whether you hate your profession or just your job or locale. How portable is your profession? If it's the kind of job you can take anywhere—such as webmaster, writer, or teacher—move to a city or town that suits you and just start working. Many careers can be turned into something portable through the Internet. Are you a burnt-out secretary? Start your own secretarial services company on the web. (If there isn't a "secretary.com" yet, someone should start one!)

- Talk to your family members and see if you have their support to pursue something else. If your family members are not behind you, you might find it more difficult to pursue what you love and might have to face deep questions about your emotional support system. Sometimes leaving relationships or marriages are involved when it comes to pursuing your dreams. In assessing what you want, you may discover that all these years you've been living behind a mask or have just been going through the motions.

Reduce the Commute

One of the simplest ways to de-stress and downshift is to eliminate that stressful commute. If you live in a bedroom community and drive into an urban centre, you may be spending more than an hour each way, to and from work. Driving is stressful, and reducing the drive can reduce a lot of stress. Here are some ways to reduce your commute:

- If you spend most of your time at work on the computer or on the phone, try to negotiate telecommuting with your employer. This means being plugged into the office from home. With teleconferencing tools, there's actually little reason to go into an office these days. Your employer can save on overhead because of the office space you'll free up, and may also attract more loyal employees because of the flexibility. (And remind your employer that telecommuters do not spend their days at home watching TV!)

- Look into moving closer to work. Have you considered this? If you calculate your car expenses, gas expenses, and so on, moving within walking distance to work may be the answer. A lot of people find trading their house in the suburbs for a rental in the city makes more sense financially. Rent and no car often equal far less than a mortgage and two cars! Car rentals for weekends away and the occasional taxi still add up to less than car-lease payments, car-financing payments, car repairs, gas and maintenance, and insurance.

- If there's no way you can move, no way your employer will let you work from home, and you're working very late hours anyway, consider renting a small apartment or room within walking distance of your office. Leave the car at the office weekdays and crash in your small "city space." Drive home weekends. Of course, if this creates more stress, don't do it, but a lot of commuters are finding that a city "crash pad" has other advantages. You can offer the pad to visiting friends or relatives (hosting visitors in your home creates stress!); other family members can use the pad when they have to be in the city for extended periods of time. And sometimes marriages and long-term relationships benefit when there's a place to go for personal space or distance in high-stress times.

Reducing Car Exhaust

Reducing the commute will also help the health of our future generations. Car exhaust is making us sick. Cancer is just one of many health risks linked to motor-vehicle emissions today. Ground-level ozone is created when volatile organic compounds meet nitrogen oxides (found in emissions from burning fossil fuels), and has been associated with lung diseases and other respiratory problems. But worst of all, car exhaust leads to "Earth sickness," since it is the ground-level ozone from motor-vehicle emissions that causes both global warming and acid rain. Put the two together and the damage to the ecosystem (not to mention our health!) may be irreparable.

Reduce Your Workweek

Moving down from a five-day workweek to a four-day workweek greatly reduces stress for many. Working Tuesday to Friday, for example, eliminates work on Monday, and according to Deepak Chopra, more people (mostly men) have heart attacks Monday mornings than any other time. Monday to Thursday is another popular choice, giving you that early start to your weekend. If you're a valued employee, many employers would rather have you working four days for them than not at all. And, when they calculate the time it takes to train someone else, they find that it's more costly to replace you than give you your four-day week. You simply reduce your salary to accommodate your new workweek.

Other ways to negotiate a reduced workweek include using vacation and sick days as "Mondays off" for a year. Some executives have weeks of unused vacation time that can be used for reduced workweeks. Some employees find that being away from the office for long periods of time actually creates more stress and guilt; taking a day off each week may be one solution to this kind of "vacationitis." Another way to reduce your workweek is to see if someone else at work wants to job-share. Surveys show that most people would trade in full-time hours for part-time hours if they could have job security. The *Miami Herald* proved the point by allowing a very stressed-out female reporter to share her job with another very stressed-out female reporter. The result was that the two less stressed and very happy reporters produced the best work of *all* the reporters.

Renegotiate Vacation Time and Leave

A study done by the American Psychosomatic Society on 12,338 men aged 35–57 found that men who took annual vacations were 21 percent less likely to die during the 16-year study period than non-vacationers and 32 percent less likely to die of coronary heart disease. This is not at all surprising. Two weeks' holiday is not enough vacation time for the average person. European companies routinely offer six weeks' vacation. When you renegotiate your vacation package, offer to combine paid vacation with unpaid leave. Surveys show that most people would gladly take unpaid vacation time if they were guaranteed job security.

A more dramatic move is to look into taking sabbatical leave. This means taking a year off for "personal reasons" (stress reduction, mental health, etc.), without pay, and returning to work the next year. Many people would take a year off if they could be guaranteed their job back upon their return. Sabbatical leave is offered to some professionals, such as teachers and tenured professors at universities, but there's no reason why it should not be an option for other working people. The payoff for cashing in some retirement funds to finance your year off comes in the form of your rejuvenation.

Slowing Down Your Life

A lot of the busyness in our lives is caused by us: we leave people too many ways to communicate with us; we try to get too many things done in the time off we have. There are ways to slow down the fast pace.

Reducing e-stress

Now that I've preached the benefits of telecommuting to you, many of you might want even more technology in your life—but let me assure you, this would only add to your stress. For most people, e-mail, voice mail, cellphones, fax machines, pagers, and the host of technology that is part of our lives have only lengthened our workdays and given us less time to ourselves. Twenty-five years ago, when you called someone who wasn't home, the phone rang many times and that was it. There was not an onus on the person called to return your call (no call would have been registered); the onus was on the caller to call back if she or he really needed to get in touch. But with voice mail, the onus is on the person called to return the call or, with the advent of Call Waiting, to answer numerous calls simultaneously. Today, to avoid phone calls, we require even more technology lest we appear to be anti-social by screening our calls. The greater access to communication that technology provides makes our "to do" lists much longer. And if you've made the mistake of subscribing to listservs, you could become bombarded with e-mails—as many as hundreds per day. The benefits and burden of technology increase with electronic organizers, Palm or Blackberry PDAs (personal digital assistants), laptops, and so forth. Even watching television has become infinitely more complicated with complex remotes that not only power the VCR and stereo system, but can rewire your house!

All this translates into *e-stress*. Part of e-stress is the learning curve. Learning to master the new technological toy can wreak havoc on the central nervous system of many. And the learning, it seems, never ends, as new gadgets keep being introduced that make the old gadgets obsolete. New versions of e-mail and fax software are also ever-problematic.

Another part of e-stress is the lack of privacy. With so many ways to be contacted, you have no safe haven that's communication-free. There is also the problem of being forced to listen to someone else's private life in public places thanks to overly loud cellphone conversations. We've all had those moments when we've glared at someone because we *really* didn't need to know about their mother's friend's colonoscopy! Each new mode of communication brings a new responsibility to reply. Experts call this "multitasking madness."

All the "e's" in your life interfere with normal communication. When you're e-mailing with one hand, talking on the phone with the other, and feeling your pager go off in the same instant, how much focused communication can you deliver? The first step in turning down the e-stress is to look at all the ways you're plugged in each day. Ask yourself these questions:

- How many phone lines do you have?
- How do you receive the Internet? If it's via cable or dedicated line, you're never "off."
- How many ways can people reach you?
- How many messages do you receive through each mode of communication? Count everything: e-mail to your office, e-mail to your home, phone messages to your cellphone and office phone, your voice mail, and so on.
- Does e-mail enhance your personal relationships or detract from them? For example, do you find yourself feeling isolated in spite of all the ways you can

contact people? Does your life partner spend his or her time with you at home … or with his or her computer? Do your children spend quality time at home or do they spend all of their time online or playing video and computer games? A 2000 Stanford University study on the societal impact of the Internet found that Internet use caused social isolation; this conclusion confirmed the findings of a 1998 study by researchers at Carnegie Mellon University.

The above questions are designed to help you evaluate the impact of the e's in your life. Reducing e-stress involves redesigning the technology in your life to work *for* you rather than *against* you. By implementing just one of the following steps, you can help reduce e-stress:

Set Up Unplugged Time.
Make a decision to be unplugged at certain times—such as after 6:00 p.m. and on weekends. You can even indicate your unplugged zone on your outgoing voice mail: "Hi. You've reached Dale at 555-5555. I check my voice mail between nine and six each day. At other times, I cannot be reached." Turn off your computer after 6:00 p.m., too, and do not check e-mail beyond a certain time. You can also set up automatic e-mail responses that tell people you're away, busy, not answering, and so on.

Use Your Cellphone Only in Case of Emergency.
Use your cellphone for outgoing emergency calls only in case of accident or something unexpected. Don't give out the number to anyone other than very close family members, and don't turn the cellphone on unless you're in an emergency situation. If you have voice mail and e-mail, people don't really need to reach you by cellphone. Don't subscribe to a message service on your cellphone, either. That way, no one can leave messages.

Limit Your Gadgets.
If you've survived this long without a Palm or Blackberry device, do you *really* need one? In other words, the more stuff you buy, the more you'll use and the less time you'll have.

Limit Your Surfing Time.
If you're searching for information about a topic on the Internet (such as stress!), you can be at your computer for days. Give yourself a limited amount of time for research, and say (as I do), "I've done the best I can with the time I have."

Limit the Messages You Save.
Try to write down the information as you get it and erase it. Otherwise, you'll spend too much time reading or listening to old messages.

Eliminate Phone Tag.
You can eliminate phone tag by leaving a specific message with specific instructions: for example, "Hi George, this is Su Lin. I will see you this Thursday, at 1:00 p.m., in front of the Coffee Mill, unless I hear otherwise." (Now George knows that he doesn't have to confirm the meeting—there's no need for another round of phone tag!)

Eliminate Energy Drains

As discussed in Chapter 4, many energy drains come in the form of people. When you're surrounded by people who take energy from you rather than give you energy in the form of support, the result is more stress in your life. But energy drains can also come from other sources, such as unmet needs in your home environment. Do you have broken appliances, car repairs that haven't been done, a wardrobe you hate, cluttered closets and rooms, or unpleasant surroundings? A home that isn't decorated in a way that pleases you makes you feel as though you don't want to be there. Plants, paint, covers for ugly furniture, and a few things on the wall often make the difference between a barren and dank home or office and a cozy and beautiful one. See the "Self-Care" section in Chapter 11 for more on the little things in life that make huge differences in your stress quotient.

Energy drains also come from procrastinating and overbooking yourself. We will procrastinate over things we really don't want to do—such as taxes. We overbook ourselves when we're afraid of saying no. Every article and book on stress management has those trite three words of advice: "Just say no." The problem is, few people will ever say it. Instead of a simple "no," try: "Let me check my schedule and see if I'm already committed." Then, "Sorry, looks like I'm committed elsewhere," or if it's a task, "I've got a deadline on that date for something of equal importance."

Finally, we drain ourselves of energy simply by doing too much and expecting too much from ourselves. When possible, hire someone to do the things you can't or don't want to do. When you're overworked at the office, subbing out one or two projects to a freelancer may be an ideal solution. If you don't think your employer will pay for the freelancer, have you considered subbing out the dreaded task on the sly and paying for it out of your own pocket? The job security, perceived "good performance," and the weight off your shoulders might be worth a couple of hundred bucks. And at home, have you considered hiring someone to do any of the following:

- Clean your house or apartment
- De-clutter your house by going through closets, filing things, and so on
- Organize your tax receipts
- Garden and/or take care of your lawn

Reduce Your Snail Mail and Plastic

Mail is stressful. How many of you have what I call "that dining-room table problem"? Does your mail get sorted and piled on the dining-room table night after night, to the point where the surface of the table disappears and you can never have company because that would mean sorting your mail? If so, you probably have too much unnecessary mail. Calling companies and requesting your name to be removed from mailing lists is often just *another* thing we have to do; so it doesn't get done. The easiest way to reduce the mail that comes inside your door is to place a garbage can or recycling bin right by your mailbox so you can sort the mail outside the house. All flyers and direct mailings (people asking for donations or selling new products, credit cards, or services) go immediately into the garbage. Don't even open them! Postcards, thank-you notes, and so on should get read on the spot, but unless you feel some dire need to save them, toss them out, too.

The next task is going through your bills and figuring out what can get paid by phone or online. Can you request a stop on snail-mail bills and ask for e-mail billings? Can you arrange to have bills paid automatically by credit or debit card and just get notice of monthly payments (such as utilities) on your credit card bill or bank statement?

As for the plastic, so much mail and stress is generated by credit cards, it's amazing. If you have too many credit cards, you're probably spending more than you can afford and accumulating massive debts. The best credit cards to have are cards that give you something in return—such as frequent flyer miles. Pick one card—*and fly with it*! Or, pick two, one for personal use and one for business use. All your department store cards (and the various loyalty programs attached to them, which can mean more cards)—toss them. Whenever I'm asked if I want to be a "member" of a club that would give me something useless for free when I spend $500 at that one store, I just say, "No thanks."

Before you cut up the cards you're not using, be sure to pay the account in full and tell the credit card company that you're *closing* your account.

And finally, try to reduce your newspaper and magazine clutter by getting a few of them online. Most daily papers are now online, for example, or at least the local information you need from them is.

Restructure Your Finances

Debt is stressful. And feeling the pressure of needing to save for retirement can also be stressful. While reducing your plastic is one small way to restructure your finances, other ways involve restructuring *your life* so that you're financing as little as possible. Here are some ways to do that:

Get Rid of Your Mortgage.
If your house is mortgaged to the hilt or in need of expensive renovations that you can't afford, that's stressful. Many people find that selling the "money pit" house and buying or renting something cheaper eliminates a lot of debt and stress.

Get Rid of Your Car.
If you're a two-car family, try living with only one car. If you're a one-car family, getting rid of the car is usually only possible in large urban centres with good public transit. Try living car-free for a year and see if it makes a difference financially. Gas, repairs, insurance, tickets, parking, and car payments really add up.

Use Retirement Funds to Pay Off Credit Card Debts or Other Nagging Debts.
Your retirement savings don't have to be used just for retirement. You're saving your money to help yourself in the future. Maybe this is the time to use some of that money. Get rid of those high-interest debts once and for all. The money you save by not paying interest can go back into your savings account.

Resist the Pressure to Play the Market.
Fund management companies may pressure you to invest your money in high-risk stocks or high-risk money market accounts, tempting you with high returns. You can certainly make money on these ventures, but you can lose your money, too. If you can't afford to lose, you may not want to play. Keeping your money in guaranteed interest accounts or lower-interest, less volatile investment accounts may give you peace of mind—something perhaps more valuable than a piece of the action! The

time and effort spent checking the stock market, worrying about the stock market, and so on can add up to a lot of wasted energy. Getting your time back from the stock market may be more valuable than the stock itself.

Slowing Down Your Kids

I spend each weekend chauffeuring my children to at least four different birthday parties as well as hockey, soccer, swimming, and karate. In between, I'm running to Toys "R" Us or Winners trying to grab cheap gifts that don't look cheap. The gifts are getting more lavish every year because I'm trying to "match" the gifts my own children receive from their friends. I reached my wit's end one day when my son came back from a party crying because his gift was refused by the birthday boy, who told him that his parents must be pretty "poor" and that he didn't need "this crappy present" (out of the mouth of an eight-year-old). The birthday boy's mother was horrified and apologized to my son and later to me, but the materialism that kids today expect is producing spoiled, rotten brats—even when the parents don't spoil them.

One of the chief causes of stress for many is what's involved these days in raising kids. The onslaught of media and advertisements from all sides is creating the perceived obligation, on the part of parents, to give their children more stuff than they actually need or want. And beyond the stuff, the variety of activities for children in suburban or affluent communities is staggering. And a lot of all this is unnecessary. Children need love, roots, and wings. They don't need to be booked up every day of the week with "play dates," various lessons, and an endless string of lavish birthday parties hosted by parents trying to outdo one another in themes, gifts, or entertainment. The more stuff you involve your children in, the more running around you have to do, the more stressed and tired the child gets (not to mention you!), and the less quality time you have to spend with your children. Here are a few tips I've mined from parents who have downshifted their children.

Limit the Lessons.
Your child does not need to be occupied with a different sport or art form every night of the week. If you want to expose your child to variety, try one different thing each school term until something sticks. One team sport or activity during the week is just fine. This will greatly reduce the amount of running around you and your family do, which will pay off in more quality family time.

Stop the Birthday Insanity.

These birthday survival tips are more doable or practical for some parents than others. But take a look:

- When your child reaches an age of "understanding," consider the gift of charity for the next birthday party he or she attends. Donate an affordable amount (say, $10) to a children's charity in the name of the birthday boy or girl. That's your gift. No more last-minute gift-shopping madness for a kid you don't know who already has everything! When it's your turn to host a birthday party, request "no gifts" but welcome donations in your children's charity of choice. This will reduce the toy clutter, the greed factor, and the inequality factor (when some children give expensive presents and others cheaper ones, the social dynamics become nightmarish all around). Reserve gift-giving for the family party you have for your child, and impress upon him or her that the "kids' party" is a time for having fun with friends, not for collecting material possessions.

- Limit the party size. Most parents agree that "eight is enough." Eight children or less is a manageable size. By limiting the number of guests, you can limit your costs and the amount of gifts your child receives. Entertain 1970s style with hot dogs or pizza, a cake, and some creative party games. Don't feel pressured to take the kids on some lavish outing.

- Reduce and reuse party gifts. Allow your child to choose a few gifts to keep and a few gifts to donate. You can use gifts from the "donate" pile for other parties, or you can give them all away to children's charities.

Living Child-Free

If you are delaying having children until your career is more settled or until you feel more financially secure, have you considered the option of *not* having a child at all?

In the past, a child-free lifestyle was often a political decision for many couples. During the 1950s and 1960s, many couples chose not to have children because they feared a nuclear holocaust. By the 1970s, the issue of overpopulation became the motivating factor in the choice. Yet by the 1980s, the option became unpopular. This is a pity, considering what a liberating option it can be. Obviously, you'll need to review your original reasons for wanting children before you make this choice. You might want to talk to child-free people to see if they regret the choice. Having and raising children is one of the most stressful experiences in life. As an author of many women's health books, I can tell you that several women have said to me, "If I knew how hard raising children would be, I wouldn't have chosen it."

Remember, parenting is a selfless, largely self-sacrificing job. Choosing a child-free lifestyle may be an appealing option in an economically turbulent and difficult world.

Some of the traditional reasons for having children were purely economic. Children, many people thought, guaranteed financial security in old age. Today, with so many college-educated adults living at home because they cannot get jobs, the economic benefits of progeny are no longer visible. And you'll find that most senior-age parents of financially successful children today don't want to be a financial burden and will choose to be independent as long as they can.

Another traditional reason for having children was fear of loneliness in one's old age. But take comfort: fifteen years from now, the majority of the population will be over 65, but the child-free among them needn't be lonely. Child-free living offers the following benefits:

Freedom.
You may have the time and extra money down the road to do all the things you've dreamed of: going back to school for that second degree, buying a vacation home, travelling, early retirement, or whatever you want.

Control of Your Life.
When you have children, you lose a certain control over your own life, as you become entangled in the precarious nature of parenting a child who lives on planet Earth. Children can have lots of problems: they may have difficulty at school; they get sick; they have accidents; they get in trouble; they get pregnant; and so on. Being a parent never stops.

Self-expansion.
You'll have the time to explore parts of yourself that you never knew existed, because you'll have time to *yourself*. You'll have the time to gain insights into your life, your gifts, your talents, your interests, and your desires.

9 HANDS-ON HEALING

All ancient non-Western cultures, whether in native North America, India, China, or Japan, have believed that there are two fundamental aspects to the human body. There is the actual physical shell (clinically called the corporeal body), which makes cells, blood, tissue, and so on, and then there is an energy flow that makes the physical body come alive. This is known as the *life force* or *life energy*. In fact, this force has been so central to the view of human function that each non-Western culture has a word for it. In China, it is called *qi* (pronounced "chee"); in India it's called *prana*; in Japan it's called *ki*; while the ancient Greeks called it *pneuma,* which has become a prefix used in medical terminology denoting breath and lungs.

Today, Western medicine concentrates on the corporeal body and does not recognize that we have a life force. In contrast, in ancient traditional medicine, it is thought that the life force heals the corporeal body, not the other way around!

Non-Western healers look upon the parts of the body as "windows" into or "maps" of the body's health. In China, the ears are a complex map, each of its points representing a different organ and part of the psyche. In reflexology, a "reading" of the feet can tell us much about the rest of the body and spirit. In the Ayerveda, the tongue is read, while other traditions read the iris of the eyes, and so on. Western medicine doesn't do this. Instead it looks at the individual parts of the body for symptoms of a disease and treats each part separately. Let's say you notice blurred vision. You might go to an eye doctor and be given a prescription for glasses and sent on your way. But if you were to go to a Chinese-medicine doctor, you would be told that the degeneration of your eyes points to an unhealthy liver. To the Chinese, the eyes are a direct window into the liver. (Interestingly, it is the eyes that turn yellow when you're jaundiced.) Instead of giving you a simple prescription for glasses, the Chinese healer will look into deeper causes of this liver imbalance in the body. You'll be asked about your personal relationships, your diet, your emotional well-being, and your job. Your treatment may involve a host of dietary changes, stress-relieving exercises, and herbal remedies. An Ayervedic doctor may use the tongue to diagnosis the same liver imbalance, but the approach is the same. You'll be asked about your diet, lifestyle, work habits, and so on. In other words, the body is not seen as separate from the self. To a non-Western healer, what makes us who we are basically has to do with our individual personalities and our societal roles. Who we marry, where we work, and how we feel about those things are just as important as our visual problems.

Energy healing is one of the most ancient forms of healing. It can involve therapeutic touch or healing touch, techniques that are considered to be forms of biofield therapy. Energy healers will use their hands to help guide your life force energy. The hands may rest on the body or just close to the body, not actually touching it. Energy healing is used to reduce pain and inflammation, improve sleep patterns and appetite, and reduce stress. Energy healing, supported by the American Holistic Nurses Association, has been incorporated into conventional nursing techniques with good results. Typically, the healer will move loosely cupped hands in a symmetric fashion on your body, sensing cold, heat, or vibration. The healer's hands are then placed over areas where the life force energy is not in balance in order to restore and regulate the energy flow.

Therapies that help to move or stimulate the life force energy include the following:

• Healing touch

• Huna

• Mari-el

• Qi gong

• Reiki

• Therapeutic touch

All forms of hands-on healing work in some way with the life force energy. This chapter outlines some of the forms of hands-on healing that can greatly reduce both physical and emotional stress.

Massage

> When my insurance plan started to cover massage, I went for my first real massage. I couldn't believe how great I felt afterwards, and now I go once a month and find a lot of my little health problems have disappeared: headaches, back pain, and so on. Curiously, even an allergy has improved. My massage therapist told me that when we are stressed, our bodies can literally "retain" emotions and stress in certain places, which is why certain parts of our bodies may feel very tender when they are "worked" compared to other spots. When the tissue is worked and manipulated and we release stress and toxins, all kinds of problems can be solved.

For many, stress relief is at their fingertips! Massage therapy can be beneficial whether you're receiving the massage from your spouse or a massage therapist trained in any one of dozens of techniques, from shiatsu to Swedish massage. In the East, massage was extensively written about in *The Yellow Emperor's Classic of Internal Medicine*, published in 2700 BC (this text frames the entire Chinese medicine tradition). In Chinese medicine, massage is recommended as a treatment for a variety of illnesses.

Swedish massage, the method Westerners are most familiar with, was developed in the 19th century by the Swedish doctor and poet Per Henrik, who borrowed techniques from ancient Egypt, China, and Rome.

It is out of shiatsu in the East and Swedish massage in the West that the many forms of massage used today were developed. While the philosophies and styles differ in each tradition, they share a common goal: to mobilize the natural healing properties of the body and thereby maintain or restore optimal health. Shiatsu-inspired massage focuses on balancing the life force energy. Swedish-inspired massage works on a more physiological principle: to relax muscles in order to improve blood flow throughout connective tissues and ultimately strengthen the cardiovascular system.

But no matter what kind of massage you have, they all use gliding and kneading techniques along with deep circular movements and vibrations to relax muscles, improve circulation, and increase mobility. Massage is known to help relieve stress and often muscle and joint pain. In fact, a number of employers cover massage therapy on their health plans. Massage is becoming so popular that the number of licensed massage therapists enrolled in the American Message Therapy Association has grown from 1,200 in 1983 to more than 38,000 today.

Massage is more technically referred to as soft-tissue manipulation. Its benefits include the following.

- Improved circulation
- Improved lymphatic system
- Faster recovery from musculoskeletal injuries
- Soothed aches and pains
- Reduced edema (water retention)
- Reduced anxiety

Types of massage include the following:

- Deep-tissue massage
- Manual lymph drainage
- Neuromuscular massage
- Sports massage
- Swedish massage

Chiropracty

The word *chiropractic* comes from the Greek words "chiro" and "prakrikos," meaning "done by hand." The tradition of chiropractic was perfected in the late 1800s by Daniel David Palmer of Port Perry, Ontario. A self-taught healer, he eventually established a practice in Iowa. He believed that all drugs are harmful and that disease is caused by vertebrae impinging on spinal nerves.

Chiropractors believe that the brain sends energy to every organ along the nerves that run through the spinal cord. When the vertebrae of the spinal column get displaced through stress, poor posture, and so on, normal nerve transmission is interfered with or blocked. These interferences are known as *subluxations*. In order to cure disease in the body, the chiropractor must remove blockages through adjustments—quick thrusts, massages, and pressures along the spinal column, which move the spinal vertebrae back to normal positions.

Sometimes adjustments involve manipulating the head and extremities (elbows, ankles, knees). This is mostly done by hand, but chiropractors also use special devices to aid them in treatment. A chiropractor will take your medical history, do a general physical examination, and perhaps x-ray your spine to look for malalignments.

Osteopathic Manipulation

Osteopathic manipulation is a hands-on healing technique utilized by an osteopathic practitioner. It involves many of the same kinds of hands-on diagnostic approaches used by a family doctor (pressing various points to gauge whether there's pain, difficulty breathing, etc.), but it also involves much more attention to things like your posture and gait (the way you walk), overall flexibility and mobility, straightness of the spine, and so on. An osteopath will carefully examine your skin, too, looking for fluid retention, muscular changes, temperature variations, and tenderness. The osteopath will then use hands-on healing techniques to manipulate and stimulate muscles, circulation, and so forth. These may be combined with standard medical treatment in certain cases, but osteopathic manipulation tends to work well to relieve the physical symptoms of stress. One of the most common forms of osteopathic manipulation is *postural drainage*, a technique used to mechanically unplug fluid blocks in the body to promote blood circulation.

Pressure Point Therapy

Pressure point therapy involves using the fingertips to apply pressure to pressure points on the body; it is believed to reduce stress, pain, and other physical symptoms of stress or other ailments. There are several different kinds of pressure point therapy. Acupuncture, reflexology, and shiatsu are three of the more well-known kinds of pressure point therapy.

Acupuncture

Acupuncture is an ancient Chinese healing art that aims to restore the smooth flow of life energy (*qi*) in your body. Acupuncturists believe that your qi can be accessed from various points on your body—your ear, for example—and that each point is linked to a specific organ. Depending on your physical health, an acupuncturist will use a fine needle on a very specific point to restore qi to various organs. Each of the roughly 2,000 points on your body has a specific therapeutic effect when stimulated. Acupuncture can relieve many of the physical symptoms and ailments caused by stress; it's now believed that acupuncture stimulates the release of endorphins, which is why it is effective in reducing stress, anxiety, pain, and so forth.

Reflexology

Western reflexology was developed by American ear, nose, and throat specialist Dr. William Fitzgerald, who talked about reflexology as "zone therapy." In fact, reflexology has been practised in several cultures, including Egypt, India, Africa, China, and Japan. Like most Eastern healing arts, reflexology aims to release the flow of energy through the body along its various pathways. When this energy is trapped for some reason, illness can result. When the energy is released, the body can begin to heal itself. A reflexologist views the foot as a microcosm of the entire body. Individual reference points or reflex areas on the foot correspond to all major organs, glands, and parts of the body. Applying pressure to a specific area of the foot stimulates the movement of energy to the corresponding body part, easing pain and tension and restoring the body's life force energy.

Shiatsu

A shiatsu healer will travel the length of each energy pathway (also called meridian), applying thumb pressure to successive points along the way. The aim is to stimulate acupressure points while giving you some of the therapist's own life energy. In barefoot shiatsu, the healer uses his or her foot instead of hand to apply pressure. Jin shin jyutsu and jin shin do are other pressure point therapies similar to acupuncture.

Working Your Own Pressure Points

You can relieve stress with your own hands, too. Here are some simple pressure point exercises you can try:

- With the thumb of one hand, slowly work your way across the palm of the other hand, from the base of the little finger to the base of the index finger. Then rub the center of your palm with your thumb. Push on this point. This will calm your nervous system. Repeat this using the other hand.

- To relieve a headache, grasp the flesh at the base of one thumb with the opposite index finger and thumb. Squeeze gently and massage the tissue in a circular motion. Then pinch each fingertip. Switch to the other hand.

- For general stress relief, find sore pressure points on your feet and ankles. Gently press your thumb into each sore point and massage it. The tender areas are signs of stress in particular parts of your body. By working them, you're relieving the stress and tension in the various organs, glands, and tissues. You can also apply pressure with bunched and extended fingers, the knuckles, the heel of the hand, or a gripping motion.

- Use the above technique for self-massage on the hands, too, looking for tender points on the palms and wrists.
- Use the above technique to self-massage the ears. Feel for tender spots on the flesh of the ears and work each one with vigorous massage. Within about four minutes the ears will get very hot.

Postural Re-Education Strategies

Postural re-education is another popular form of hands-on healing. It involves the use of touch to guide your body into better posture and alignment and is similar in some ways to chiropractic healing. By learning better posture, coordination, and balance, structural and functional stress is relieved. Three of the most common postural re-education methods used in North America are the Alexander technique, the Feldenkrais method, and Trager psychophysical integration.

The Alexander Technique

The Alexander technique focuses on the repositioning of the head, neck, and shoulders. Developed by Shakespearean actor Frederick Matthias Alexander (1869–1955), it involves being verbally guided into better posture and alignment through exercises where one may be lying, sitting, standing, or walking. The purpose of these exercises is to address posture-related tension. By avoiding certain movements, you can greatly decrease back pain or back problems, improve overall health, and improve your mental health (you'll have better focus, more patience, and so on).

The Feldenkrais Method

The Feldenkrais method was developed by physicist Moshe Feldenkrais. He believed that movement, thought, speech, and feelings are reflections of self-image, and argued that when people are made aware of their habits related to motion, they can be taught to move more easily and gracefully, resulting in improved self-image and better health. A combination of verbal guidance and gentle touch is used to make you aware of customary movement patterns and possible alternatives. You can improve your stress-related symptoms and overall health if you move with more grace and awareness.

The Trager Method

The Trager method was developed by Milton Trager, M.D. (1908–97), and is often called the Trager Approach. This method involves learning the joy of movement. Practitioners of this method use their hands to direct you through exercises involving bouncing, rocking, shaking, compression, and elongation. It is believed that by using and moving your body in all the ways it *can* be moved, you can improve your mind-set, flexibility, and overall health, and reduce stress-related tension. Trager was born with a congenital spinal deformity, but through this method, he developed an athletic and graceful body.

Rolfing: Structural Integration

Developed by Ida Rolf, a biophysicist, rolfing involves realigning bad posture caused by trauma or injury. Healers who use the Rolfing technique will coax bones and muscles into proper alignment by using their thumbs, fingers, and elbows to deliver a sliding pressure to the affected area. Rolfing can cause some discomfort because it involves stretching the deep tissues sufficiently to bring the head, torso, pelvis, legs, and feet into alignment. The results, however, can be rewarding; stress can be greatly reduced or alleviated through Rolfing.

Where to Find Hands-On Healers

If you're interested in trying out one of these techniques, contact your family doctor or chiropractor for a referral. Naturopathic physicians are also a good source. The "hairdresser" rule is also a good way to locate these practitioners. Friends and family members who've had good experiences with any of these techniques are probably good resources for you as well.

When you find the practitioner in the discipline that interests you, be sure to tell him or her about any medications you're taking and medical conditions you might have. It's not recommended to seek out treatment while you have an active infection or virus, such as a cold or flu. If you have inflamed or infected tissue, an infectious disease, or a serious heart condition, or are undergoing treatment for cancer, consult your doctor before receiving any of these therapies. There is concern that some of these techniques could worsen some medical conditions.

The benefits of many of these healing techniques have not yet been proven in standard Western studies. It's important to keep in mind that when it comes to researching alternative therapies, most Western researchers don't know enough about them to design proper studies. And many of these ancient disciplines just don't lend themselves well to Western-style research, such as double-blind controlled studies. You should, however, be aware of the risks associated with alternative and complementary medicine:

- No scientific proof exists to support most of the treatments you'll be offered or to support the claims of the therapies.

- Since there is no advisory board or set of guidelines that govern non-Western practitioners, the alternative "industry" attracts quacks and charlatans; as well, costs for some therapies can be prohibitive.

- Academic credentials are all over the map in this industry. Beware of humbugs.

A Proper Back Rub

How many times have you asked someone for a back rub, only to be completely disappointed by poor technique. Now you can hand your back rubber this page. You can also show the back rubber the right way to do it, by reciprocating the favour.

Step One: Using the heels of your hands, do a long stroke starting from the buttocks and following the length of the spine (both sides of the spine).

Step Two: At the shoulders, use your thumbs to make small deep circles starting in the interior part of the shoulder blades; move up the spine into the base of the head and then down to the small of the back.

Step Three: At the base of the head, press your forefinger and middle finger into the furrows.

Repeat these steps until your recipient is relaxed.

ANTI-STRESS HERBS AND NUTRIENTS

A variety of "nerve herbs" are available over-the-counter at most drugstores and natural health food stores. An herb that is said to be "nervine" has a positive effect on the nervous system. It could be toning, relaxing, or stimulating; it could act as an antidepressant or analgesic. Food, too, contains a range of stress-busting nutrients, some of which may be missing in your diet. This chapter describes some stress-busting herbs and foods that you may not know about.

Herbs That Calm

When my mother was dying, I started to have these attacks where I couldn't breathe. My girlfriend told me about "Rescue Remedy," which she'd started using for panic attacks around the time of her divorce. When I asked my doctor about this, she didn't know what I was talking about and asked me if I wanted a prescription for Zoloft. I got the feeling that my doctor wasn't all that informed about anything natural, and decided that my girlfriend was a better source, since she had been through it. It turns out that Rescue Remedy has been around for decades in homeopathic circles. Now it's what I use to control my panic, and I'm surprised medical doctors aren't more forthcoming about natural remedies. They'd rather give you harsh drugs with side-effects.

Many people find the following herbal supplements helpful in combatting the range of emotional symptoms stress can create, such as irritability, anxiety, sleeplessness, and mild to moderate depression.

St. John's Wort.

Also known as hypericum, St. John's wort has been used as a nerve tonic in folk medicine for centuries. It's been shown to successfully treat mild to moderate depression as well as anxiety. It's been used in Germany for years as a first-line treatment for depression and is endorsed by the American Psychiatric Association. In Germany and other parts of Europe, it outsells Prozac. Since it was introduced into North America in the early 1990s, millions of North Americans have been successfully treated for depression with this herb. In the United States, sales of St. John's wort and other botanical products reached an estimated $4.3 billion dollars in 1998, according to *Nutrition Business Journal*. The herb has several benefits: it has minimal side-effects; it can be mixed with alcohol; it is non-addictive; you don't need to increase your dose for the same effect as you do with antidepressants; you can go on and off of St. John's wort as you wish, without any problem; it helps you sleep and dream; and it doesn't have any sedative effect and in fact enhances your alertness.

Kava Root.

From the black pepper family, kava (*Piper methysticum*) has been a popular herbal drink in the South Pacific for centuries. Kava grows on the islands of Polynesia and is known to calm nerves, ease stress, fatigue, and anxiety, and have an antidepressant effect. Kava can also help alleviate migraine headaches and menstrual cramps. Placebo-controlled studies conducted by the National Institute of Mental Health showed that kava significantly relieves anxiety and stress without the problem of dependency or addiction. Kava should not be combined with alcohol because it can intensify the effects of alcohol. You should check with your doctor before you combine kava with any prescription medication.

SAM-e.

Pronounced "Sammy," Sam-e is another natural compound shown to help alleviate anxiety and mild depression. Since it was introduced in the United States in March 1999, it has outsold St. John's wort. Sam-e has been shown to relieve joint pain and improve liver function, which makes it popular with arthritis sufferers. Sam-e stands for S-adenosylmethionine, a compound made by the body's cells. Studies done in Italy during the 1970s documented Sam-e's effectiveness as an antidepressant; recent U.S. studies confirm those results. Some people have reported hot, itchy ears as a side-effect.

Ginkgo.

A common herb in Chinese medicine, ginkgo is used to treat a variety of ailments. It can improve memory, and some studies show that it can boost the effectiveness of antidepressant medications.

Valerian Root.

Like kava root, valerian root works as an anti-anxiety agent. It also alleviates insomnia. Valerian root in combination with passion flower, oatstraw, or chamomile is very relaxing, toning, and restorative.

Ginseng.

Ginseng helps you adapt to stress (physical or psychological). It is also considered to boost the immune system.

Astragalus.

Similar to ginseng, this Chinese herb helps you adapt to stress by strengthening the immune system.

Flower Power

Bach flower remedies can be counted among today's most popular natural emotional "rescues." These remedies comprise 38 homeopathically prepared plant and flower liquid extracts. Each flower remedy is designed to treat a different emotion. Dr. Edward Bach invented this healing tradition in the 1930s (during a time of extreme economic and social misery). Bach classified emotions according to seven major groups (e.g., fear, uncertainty, loneliness), identifying 38 different emotional states and creating 38 corresponding flower remedies. These remedies work through homeopathic principles, stimulating the body's own capacity to heal itself. The flower remedies are made available as a liquid, to which brandy is added as a preservative. Taking the remedy involves diluting two drops of the pure liquid in 2 tablespoons/30 mL of mineral water. You then take four drops of the dilution orally four times a day. You can also put two drops of the pure remedy into a glass of water, and just sip it throughout the day.

Rescue Remedy

Rescue Remedy is a combination of five Bach flower remedies: Cherry Plum, Clematis, Impatiens, Rock Rose, and Star of Bethlehem. This combination works well for people who suffer from panic attacks or anxiety, and is designed to be taken pure, or "neat," from the bottle. You don't need to buy all the Bach flower remedies and combine them yourself, as Rescue Remedy comes premixed. People can either take four drops of Rescue Remedy at once, orally, or dilute four drops in a glass of water and drink. Rescue Remedy reportedly works very quickly to calm the emotions.

The 38 Bach Flower Remedies

The following is a complete list of the Bach flower remedies and the corresponding emotional states that they help to calm or quell.

1. Agrimony – mental torture behind a cheerful face
2. Aspen – fear of unknown things
3. Beech – intolerance
4. Centaury – the inability to say "no"
5. Cerato – lack of trust in one's own decisions
6. Cherry Plum – fear of the mind giving way
7. Chestnut Bud – failure to learn from mistakes
8. Chicory – selfish, possessive love
9. Clematis – dreaming of the future without working in the present
10. Crab Apple – the cleansing remedy, also for self-hatred
11. Elm – overwhelmed by responsibility
12. Gentian – discouragement after a setback
13. Gorse – hopelessness and despair
14. Heather – self-centredness and self-concern
15. Holly – hatred, envy, and jealousy
16. Honeysuckle – living in the past
17. Hornbeam – procrastination, tiredness at the thought of doing something
18. Impatiens – impatience
19. Larch – lack of confidence
20. Mimulus – fear of known things
21. Mustard – deep gloom for no reason
22. Oak – the plodder who keeps going past the point of exhaustion
23. Olive – exhaustion following mental or physical effort

24. Pine – guilt

25. Red Chestnut – over-concern for the welfare of loved ones

26. Rock Rose – terror and fright

27. Rock Water – self-denial, rigidity, and self-repression

28. Scleranthus – inability to choose between alternatives

29. Star of Bethlehem – shock

30. Sweet Chestnut – extreme mental anguish, when everything has been tried and there is no light left

31. Vervain – over-enthusiasm

32. Vine – dominance and inflexibility

33. Walnut – protection from change and unwanted influences

34. Water Violet – pride and aloofness

35. White Chestnut – unwanted thoughts and mental arguments

36. Wild Oat – uncertainty over one's direction in life

37. Wild Rose – drifting, resignation, apathy

38. Willow – self-pity and resentment

Source: Dr Edward Bach Centre, **www.bachcentre.com**. Reprinted with permission, 2002.

Making Scents

Essential oils derived from plants (mostly herbs and flowers) can do wonders to relieve stress naturally; many essential oils are known for their calming and antidepressant effects. Table 10.1 shows which essential oils are used to treat specific stress ailments. All oils listed in the table can be used in a diffuser (a ceramic pot with a tea light underneath and a bowl of water on top into which the oils are dropped; a light-bulb ring also works), in a hot bath (you can drop the oils directly into the hot water), or as a massage oil (you need a "carrier" base oil such as olive, jojoba, carrot seed, grape seed, or sweet-almond). You can also mix certain oils into an unscented moisturizer and apply to your face (neroli, lavender, ylang-ylang, and rose all make excellent facial oils). Twelve drops of oil in any of these methods is the average dose. When oils are applied directly to the skin, two drops is the average. Applying any of the oils directly to the soles of the feet is a good way to feel their effectiveness faster.

TABLE 10.1 Aromatherapy for Stress Relief

To Help with Feelings of ...	Try ...
Anxiety, panic, anger, depression	*Calming scents*: bergamot, cedarwood, chamomile, clary sage, geranium, jasmine, lavender, myrrh, neroli, patchouli, rose, sage, sandalwood, tangerine, ylang ylang
Fatigue or decreased concentration	*Stimulating scents:* Basil, cedarwood, cypress, fir, frankincense, geranium, ginger, jasmine, juniper, marjoram, peppermint, rose, rosemary, rosewood, sandalwood, spruce, thyme, ylang-ylang. *To invigorate, try:* frankincense, ginger, grapefruit, juniper, pepper and rosewood.
Forgetfulness	Basil, bergamot, clove, ginger, grapefruit, lavender, lemon, cedarwood, chamomile (Roman), cypress, fir, geranium, juniper, marjoram, myrrh, orange, rose, rosemary, sandalwood, rose, ylang-ylang
Restlessness	Angelica, basil, bergamot, cedarwood, frankincense, geranium, lavender, orange, rose, rosewood, spruce, valor, ylang-ylang

To Help Combat ...	Try ...
Acne or other skin eruptions	Bergamot, cedarwood, chamomile, clary sage, eucalyptus, juniper, lavender, lemon, marjoram, tea tree oil, patchouli, rosemary, rosewood, sage, thyme (can be applied on the blotches directly)
Asthma	Cypress, eucalyptus, fir, frankincense, hyssop, lavender, lemon, marjoram, myrrh, myrtle, oregano, peppermint, ravensara, rose, rosemary, sage, thyme (can apply to pillow or over lungs/throat topically)
Backache	As a massage oil: cypress, helichrysum, peppermint
Chills, shakiness, and dizziness (when feeling panic, for example)	Ginger (apply to bottoms of feet)
Cold/flu	To clear congestion or respiratory tract, or to break a fever, apply to soles of feet and back of neck or bathe in: peppermint, eucalyptus, ginger
Constipation	Fennel, ginger, juniper, marjoram, orange, patchouli, pepper (black), rose, rosemary, sandalwood, tangerine, tarragon (can be applied as a massage oil to the lower abdomen)
Diarrhea	Geranium, ginger, tea tree, myrrh, myrtle, peppermint, sandalwood, spearmint
Headaches	Clove, eucalyptus, frankincense, lavender, marjoram, peppermint, rosemary (apply to temples, back of neck and forehead)
Heart pounding	Orange, lavender, melissa, peppermint, ylang-ylang
Insomnia	Angelica, clary sage, cypress, lavender, lemon, marjoram, myrtle, orange, ravensara, rosemary, sandalwood, ylang-ylang (bathe in any of these before bed or drop on pillow)
Joint and muscle pain	Birch, ginger, nutmeg, rosemary, juniper, nutmeg, spruce
Nausea	Clove, ginger, juniper, lavender, nutmeg, peppermint, rosewood, spearmint, tarragon (put on a cotton ball and inhale, or put behind the ears)

Note: In general, the following essential oils are considered essential for the female system in terms of balancing hormones and offsetting a number of discomforts: bergamot, clary sage, clove, fennel, geranium, nutmeg, sage, ylang-ylang.

Sources: Connie Higley, Alan Higley, and Pat Leatham, *Aromatherapy A–Z* (Carlsbad, CA: Hay House, 1998); Alison Wood, "Common Scents," in *Look Good Feel Better* (Canadian Cosmetic, Toiletry & Fragrance Association Foundation, 2001), 21.

Herbs for the Heart

If stress is causing you to experience heart palpitations or if you're concerned about the effects of stress on your heart, the following nutrients are good for strengthening or nourishing the heart:

- Wheat germ oil. One or more tablespoons/15 mL daily.
- Vitamin E oil. One or more tablespoons/15 mL daily.
- Flaxseed (*Linum usitatissimum*), also known as linseed, is considered the best heart oil—but only if it is absolutely fresh and taken uncooked. One to 3 teaspoons/5–15 mL of flaxseed oil first thing in the morning is recommended. You can also grind the seeds and sprinkle them on cereals or salads. You can soak flaxseeds in water and drink the whole thing first thing in the morning.
- Other heart protective oils can be found in the fresh-pressed oils of borage seed or black currant seed.
- Other essential fatty acids can be found in plantain, lamb's quarter, or amaranth.
- Hawthorn berry tincture. Take 25–40 drops of the berry tincture up to four times a day. Expect results no sooner than 6–8 weeks.
- Seaweed
- Carotene-rich foods. Look for bright-coloured fruits and vegetables. The richer the colour, the richer they are in carotene.
- Garlic (*Allium sativum*). Greatest heart benefits come from eating it raw, but you can also purchase deodorized caplets.
- Lemon balm. Steep a handful of fresh leaves in a glass of white wine for an hour or so and drink it with dinner. Or make lemon balm vinegar to use on your salads.
- Dandelion root tincture. Use 10–15 drops with meals.
- Ginseng (*Panax quinquefolium*). Chew on the root or use 5–40 drops of tincture.
- Motherwort (*Leonurus cardiaca*). Use a tincture of the flowering tops, 5–15 drops several times a day as needed.

Herbs That Calm the Heart

As discussed in Chapter 1, stress can cause panic attacks and heart palpitations. The following herbs reportedly calm the heart.

- Rose flower essence
- Hawthorn (Crataegus). Try 25–40 drops up to four times a day. Slow acting, it requires about a month of use before you see results.
- Motherwort tincture. Take 10–20 drops with meals and before bed or 25–50 drops for immediate relief.
- Valerian root, as a tea or tincture
- Ginger root tea, hot or cold
- A piece of real licorice root to slow palpitations

Lowering Your Risk of Heart Attack or Stroke

Blood thinners, such as aspirin, can reduce the incidence of stroke or heart attack. A daily spoonful of vinegar made from the leaves, buds, and/or flowers of any of the following herbs gives you the same health benefits as aspirin, but also helps calcium absorption and improves your digestion. Do not take blood-thinning herbs if you are bleeding heavily or require surgery.

- Alfalfa
- Birch
- Sweet clover
- Bedstraw
- Poplar
- Red clover
- Willow
- Wintergreen
- Black haw (viburnum). As a tincture, a 25-drop dose as needed.

To Lower Blood Pressure

- **Hawthorn**. As a tincture, 10–20 drops three times daily.
- **Motherwort**. As a tincture, 10–20 drops three times daily.
- **Dandelion root**. As a tincture, 10–15 drops with meals.

- **Potassium**. Eighty to 85 percent of people who eat six portions of potassium-rich foods daily will reduce their need for blood-pressure–lowering medication by half or more.

- **Raw garlic.** Just 1/2 to 1 clove of raw garlic a day can dramatically reduce your blood pressure. Mince it raw into a variety of dishes, including eggs, rice, and potatoes.

- **Ginseng**

- **Seaweed**

Gut Reactions

Stress can seriously interfere with digestion. The following spices can aid digestion anytime, but especially during high-stress periods:

- **Coriander.** Eases gases and works to tone the digestive system. Use powdered or whole seed, or garnish with fresh leaves (cilantro).

- **Cardamom.** Reduces the mucus-forming effects of dairy products. Use powdered or whole seeds.

- **Turmeric.** Generally improves metabolism and helps you digest proteins. Use the root ground. (Gives dishes a yellowish colour and can stain clothes and china.)

- **Black pepper.** Stimulates appetite and helps you digest dairy products. Use freshly ground.

- **Cumin.** Helps reduce gases and generally tones the digestive system. Use seeds whole or powdered.

- **Fennel.** Helps prevent gas. Chew the seeds after a meal, or cook them with vegetables that tend to produce gas. Use whole or powdered.

- **Ginger.** Aids digestion and respiration. Also helps to relieve gas, constipation, and indigestion. Use root fresh or dried. (Note: ginger can aggravate bleeding ulcers.)

- **Cinnamon.** Naturally cleanses your digestive system. Use powdered, in sticks, or in pieces.

- **Nutmeg.** Helps your body absorb nutrients from food, but should be used sparingly.

- **Clove.** Helps your body absorb nutrients. Use whole or ground.

- **Cayenne.** Helps to simulate your digestive juices and is known for having a "cleansing action" within the large intestine. Helps to relieve that feeling of fullness after a heavy meal.

- **Licorice root.** Take 2–4 capsules after meals as a general digestive aid.

Reducing Stress through Food

We now know that a variety of daily nutrients can help to regulate our stress levels and our moods. Tryptophan, for example, which is found in milk and other dairy products, helps our bodies build neurotransmitters, such as serotonin.

The B vitamins are also important for our mental health. Vitamin B_{12} is crucial for good general health, while other B-complex vitamins (thiamine, riboflavin, niacin, pyridoxine, pantothenic acid, and biotin) are essential for brain function, enabling us to be cognizant and alert. You'll find the B vitamins in lean meats, whole grains, liver, seeds, nuts, wheat germ, and dairy products. Folate (a.k.a. folic acid) is particularly important for a healthy mood. It's found in liver, eggs, leafy greens, yeast, legumes, whole grains, nuts, fruits (bananas, orange juice, grapefruit juice), vegetables (broccoli, spinach, asparagus, Brussels sprouts). If you aren't eating enough "brain foods," you are more prone to stress, anxiety, and depression.

Calcium and magnesium help your brain properly transmit nerve impulses. Calcium is found in dairy products, leafy greens, eggs, and fish (particularly salmon and sardines). Magnesium-rich foods include soy, nuts, whole grains, milk, meat, and fish.

Here's a summary of all the natural sources for the various nutrients you need for mental and physical health:

Vitamin A/Beta Carotene.
Vitamin A is found in liver, fish oils, egg yolks, whole milk, butter; beta carotene (and vitamin A) is found in leafy greens, yellow and orange vegetables, and fruits. Both are depleted by coffee, alcohol, cortisone, mineral oil, fluorescent lights, liver "cleansing," excessive intake of iron, lack of protein.

Vitamin B_6.
Found in meats, poultry, fish, nuts, liver, bananas, avocados, grapes, pears, egg yolk, whole grains, legumes.

Vitamin B$_{12}$.

Found in meats, dairy products, eggs, liver, fish. Both B$_{12}$ and B$_6$ are depleted by coffee, alcohol, tobacco, sugar, raw oysters, birth control pills.

Vitamin C.

Found in citrus fruits, broccoli, green pepper, strawberries, cabbage, tomato, cantaloupe, potatoes, leafy greens. Herbal sources: rosehip, yellow dock root, raspberry leaf, red clover, hops, nettles, pine needles, dandelion greens, alfalfa, echinacea, skullcap, parsley, cayenne, paprika. Depleted by antibiotics, aspirin and other pain relievers, coffee, stress, aging, smoking, baking soda, high fever.

Vitamin D.

Found in fortified milk, butter, leafy green vegetables, egg yolk, fish oils, butter, liver, skin exposure to sunlight, shrimp. Herbal sources: none; not found in plants. Depleted by mineral oil used on the skin, frequent baths, sunscreens with SPF 8 or higher.

Vitamin E.

Found in nuts, seeds, whole grains, fish-liver oils, fresh leafy greens, kale, cabbage, asparagus. Herbal sources: alfalfa, rosehips, nettles, dang gui, watercress, dandelion, seaweed, wild seeds. Depleted by mineral oil, sulphates.

Vitamin K.

Found in leafy greens, corn and soybean oils, liver, cereals, dairy products, meats, fruits, egg yolk, blackstrap molasses. Herbal sources: nettles, alfalfa, kelp, green tea. Depleted by x-rays, radiation, air pollution, enemas, frozen foods, antibiotics, rancid fats, aspirin.

Thiamine (Vitamin B$_1$).

Found in asparagus, cauliflower, cabbage, kale, spirulina, seaweed, citrus. Herbal sources: peppermint, burdock, sage, yellow dock, alfalfa, red clover, fenugreek, raspberry leaves, nettles, catnip, watercress, yarrow, briar rose buds, rosehips.

Riboflavin (B$_2$).

Found in beans, greens, onions, seaweed, spirulina, dairy products, mushrooms. Herbal sources: peppermint, alfalfa, parsley, echinacea, yellow dock, hops, dandelion, ginseng, dulse, kelp, fenugreek.

Pyridoxine (B$_6$).
Found in baked potato with skin, broccoli, prunes, bananas, dried beans, lentils, all meats, poultry, fish.

Folic Acid (B Factor).
Found in liver, eggs, leafy greens, yeast, legumes, whole grains, nuts, fruits (bananas, orange juice, grapefruit juice), vegetables (broccoli, spinach, asparagus, Brussels sprouts). Herbal sources: nettles, alfalfa, parsley, sage, catnip, peppermint, plantain, comfrey leaves, chickweed.

Niacin (B Factor).
Found in grains, meats, nuts, and especially asparagus, spirulina, cabbage, bee pollen. Herbal sources: hops, raspberry leaf, red clover, slippery elm, echinacea, licorice, rosehips, nettles, alfalfa, parsley.

Bioflavonoids.
Found in citrus pulp and rind. Herbal sources: buckwheat greens, blue green algae, elder berries, hawthorn fruit, rosehips, horsetail, shepherd's purse.

Carotenes.
Found in carrots, cabbage, winter squash, sweet potatoes, dark leafy greens, apricots, spirulina, seaweed. Herbal sources: peppermint, yellow dock, uva ursi, parsley, alfalfa, raspberry leaves, nettles, dandelion greens, kelp, green onions, violet leaves, cayenne, paprika, lamb's quarters, sage peppermint, chickweed, horsetail, black cohosh, rosehips.

Essential Fatty Acids (EFAs).
Essential fatty acids, including GLA, omega-6, and omega-3, are found in safflower oil, wheat germ oil. Herbal sources: all wild plants contain EFAs. Commercial sources: flaxseed oil, evening primrose, black current, borage.

Boron.
Found in organic fruits, vegetables, nuts. Herbal sources: all organic weeds, including chickweed, purslane, nettles, dandelion, yellow dock.

Calcium.
Found in milk and dairy products, leafy greens, broccoli, clams, oysters, almonds, walnuts, sunflower seeds, sesame seeds (e.g., tahini), legumes, tofu, softened bones of canned fish (sardines, mackerel, salmon), seaweed, vegetables, whole grain, whey, shellfish. Herbal sources: valerian, kelp, nettles, horsetail, peppermint, sage, uva ursi,

yellow dock, chickweed, red clover, oatstraw, parsley, blackcurrent leaf, raspberry leaf, plantain leaf/seed, borage, dandelion leaf, amaranth leaves, lamb's quarter. Depleted by coffee, sugar, salt, alcohol, cortisone enemas, too much phosphorus.

Chromium.
Found in barley grass, bee pollen, prunes, nuts, mushrooms, liver, beets, whole wheat. Herbal sources: oatstraw, nettles, red clover, catnip, dulse, wild yam, yarrow, horsetail, black cohosh, licorice, echinacea, valerian, sarsaparilla. Depleted by white sugar.

Copper.
Found in liver, shellfish, nuts, legumes, water, organically grown grains, leafy greens, seaweed, bittersweet chocolate. Herbal sources: skullcap, sage, horsetail, chickweed.

Iron.
Heme iron is easily absorbed by the body; non-heme iron is not as easily absorbed, so should be taken with vitamin C. Heme iron is found in liver, meat, poultry; non-heme iron is found in dried fruit, seeds, almonds, cashews, enriched and whole grains, legumes, green leafy vegetables. Herbal sources: chickweed, kelp, burdock, catnip, horsetail, Althea root, milk thistle seed, uva ursi, dandelion leaf/root, yellow dock root, dang gui, black cohosh, echinacea, plantain leaves, sarsaparilla, nettles, peppermint, licorice, valerian, fenugreek. Depleted by coffee, black tea, enemas, alcohol, aspirin, carbonated drinks, lack of protein, too much dairy.

Magnesium.
Found in leafy greens, seaweed, nuts, whole grains, yogurt, cheese, potatoes, corn, peas, squash. Herbal sources: oatstraw, licorice, kelp, nettle, dulse, burdock, chickweed, Althea root, horsetail, sage, raspberry leaf, red clover, valerian, yellow dock, dandelion, carrot tops, parsley, evening primrose. Depleted by alcohol, chemical diuretics, enemas, antibiotics, excessive fat intake.

Manganese.
Found in seaweed and in any leaf or seed from a plant grown in healthy soil. Herbal sources: raspberry leaf, uva ursi, chickweed, milk thistle, yellow dock, ginseng, wild yam, hops, catnip, echinacea, horsetail, kelp, nettles, dandelion.

Molybdenum.
Found in organically raised dairy products, legumes, grains, leafy greens. Herbal sources: nettles, dandelion greens, sage, oatstraw, fenugreek, raspberry leaves, red clover, horsetail, chickweed, seaweed.

Nickel.
Found in chocolate, nuts, dried beans, cereals. Herbal sources: alfalfa, red clover, oatstraw, fenugreek.

Phosphorus.
Found in whole grains, seeds, nuts. Herbal sources: peppermint, yellow dock, milk thistle, fennel, hops, chickweed, nettles, dandelion, parsley, dulse, red clover. Depleted by antacids.

Potassium.
Found in bananas, celery, cabbage, peas, parsley, broccoli, peppers, carrots, potato skins, eggplant, whole grains, pears, citrus, seaweed. Herbal sources: sage, catnip, hops, dulse, peppermint, skullcap, kelp, red clover, horsetail, nettles, borage, plantain. Depleted by coffee, sugar, salt, alcohol, enemas, vomiting, diarrhea, chemical diuretics, dieting.

Selenium.
Found in dairy products, seaweed, grains, garlic, liver, kidneys, fish, shellfish. Herbal sources: catnip, milk thistle, valerian, dulse, black cohosh, ginseng, uva ursi, hops, echinacea, kelp, raspberry leaf, rose buds, rosehips, hawthorn berries, fenugreek, sarsaparilla, yellow dock.

Silicon.
Found in unrefined grains, root vegetables, spinach, leeks. Herbal sources: horsetail, dulse, echinacea, cornsilk, burdock, oatstraw, licorice, chickweed, uva ursi, sarsaparilla.

Sulfur.
Found in eggs, dairy products, cabbage family plants, onions, garlic, parsley, watercress. Herbal sources: nettles, sage, plantain, horsetail.

Zinc.
Found in oysters, seafood, meat, liver, eggs, whole grains, wheat germ, pumpkin seeds, spirulina. Herbal sources: skullcap, sage, wild yam, chickweed, echinacea, nettles, dulse, milk thistle, sarsaparilla. Depleted by alcohol and air pollution.

Supplementing Your Diet

When we're under stress, we're usually depleted in vitamins and minerals. Most of us know that the anti-stress vitamins are vitamin C (RDI: 4–8 g) and the B vitamins, particularly cyanocobalamin, or B_{12} (RDI: 50–250 mcg); niacin, or B_3 (RDI: 50–150 mg); pyridoxine, or B_6 (RDI: 50–100 mg); and riboflavin, or B_2 (RDI: 50–100 mg). All of the B vitamins can be found in a B-complex vitamin supplement, but you should also supplement with the following: Beta-carotene, 10,000–25,000 IUs (International Units).

- Bioflavonoids, 250–500 mg
- Biotin, 150–500 mcg
- Calcium, 600–1000 mg
- Chromium, 200–400 mcg
- Copper, 2–3 mg
- Folic acid, 500–1000 mcg
- Hydrochloric acid (with meals for chronic stress), 5–10 grains
- Inositol, 500–1000 mg
- Iodine, 150–200 mcg
- Iron (menstruating women especially), 10–20 mg
- L-amino acids (e.g., L-glutamine, L-tyrosine, L-phenylalanine, L-tryptophan), 1000–1500 mg
- L-cysteine (take with vitamin C), 250–500 mg
- Magnesium (an Epsom salt bath is also magnesium), 350–600 mg
- Manganese, 5–10 mg
- Molybdenum, 300–800 mg
- PABA, 50–100 mg
- Pancreatic enzymes (after meals), 1–2 tablets
- Pantothenic acid (B_5), 500–1000 mg
- Potassium, 300–500 mg
- Pyridoxal-5-phosphate, 25–75 mg
- Selenium, 200–400 mcg
- Sulfur (check with your doctor or pharmacist about RDI)

- Superoxide dismutase (an enzyme—check with your doctor or pharmacist about RDI)
- Thiamine (B_1), 75–150 mg
- Vitamin A , 7500–15,000 IUs
- Vitamin D, 400 IUs
- Vitamin E, 400–1000 IUs
- Vitamin K, 200–400 mcg
- Water, 2–3 quarts/2–2.5 L
- Zinc, 30–60 mg

The following substances can also help with stress:

- **Gamma-aminobutyric acid (GABA).** GABA is an amino acid that is supposedly an anti-anxiety agent that may also help you to fall asleep if you suffer from sleeplessness.

- **Inositol.** Inositol is a naturally occurring antidepressant present in many foods, such as vegetables, whole grains, milk, and meat, and should be available over-the-counter.

- **Dehydroepiandrosterone (DHEA).** DHEA is a hormone produced by the adrenal glands; production declines as we age. It has been shown to improve moods and memory in certain studies, but it is not yet available in Canada.

- **Melatonin.** Melatonin is a hormone that improves sleep and helps reset the body's natural clock. It is not yet available in Canada.

- **Phosphatidylserine (PS).** PS is a phospholipid, a substance that feeds brain-cell membranes. Some studies show that it has natural antidepressant qualities.

- **Tetrahydrobiopterin (BH4).** BH4 activates enzymes that control serotonin, noradrenaline, and dopamine levels, which are all important for a stable mood. Some studies show that BH4 is an effective natural treatment for depression.

- **Phenylethylamine (PEA).** PEA is a nitrogen-containing compound found in small quantities in the brain. Studies show that it works as a natural antidepressant.

- **Rubidium.** Rubidium is a natural chemical in our bodies, belonging to the same family as lithium, potassium, and sodium. Studies show that it can work as an antidepressant.

IMPROVING TRANQUILITY

There are a number of ways to improve your overall sense of tranquility or harmony. In some cases, taking up an actual discipline, such as yoga, can dramatically improve your sense of well-being and lower your stress. In other cases, just employing some basic self-care can do wonders.

Life and Breath

In previous chapters, I discussed the non-Western concept of life force energy. The following practices use breathing to help move life force energies through the body.

Yoga

Yoga is not just about various stretches or postures; it is actually a way of life for many and part of a whole science of living known as the Ayerveda. The Ayerveda is an ancient Indian approach to health and wellness that has stood up quite well to the test of time. It's roughly 3,000 years old. According to the Ayerveda, the universe has three basic constitutions or "energies." Known as doshas, the energies are based on wind (*vata*), fire (*pitta*), and earth (*kapha*). The doshas govern our bodies, personalities, and activities. When our doshas are balanced, everything functions well, but when they are not balanced, a state of disease (dis-ease as in "not at ease") can set in. Finding the balance involves changing your diet to suit your predominant dosha.

Foods are classified as kapha, vata, or pitta, and we eat more or less of whatever we need for balance.

Yoga is a preventive health science that involves meditation and certain physical postures and exercises. Essentially, it is the "exercise" component of the Ayerveda. It involves relaxing meditation, breathing, and physical postures designed to tone and soothe your mental and physical state. Most people benefit from introductory yoga classes or even introductory videos.

Qi Gong

> When I started doing qi gong, I was dragged kicking and screaming by my girlfriend, who assured me it would change my life. I had been suffering from constipation for a long time, and we did these series of exercises based on the five Seasons (in China, there are five distinct seasons instead of four). One of the exercises was bringing qi into the lungs, which according to the Chinese organ system are linked to the colon. In the middle of the exercise, I started to have an urge to go to the bathroom and had to leave the class. My constipation never bothered me after that, and I faithfully do that particular exercise.

Every morning, all over China, people of all ages gather in parks to do their daily qi gong exercises. Pronounced "chi kung," these exercises help get your life force energy (called *qi* in Chinese) flowing and unblocked. Qi gong exercises are modelled after the movements of wildlife (such as birds or animals), of trees, and of other things in nature. The exercises have a continuous flow, rather than the stillness of a posture seen in yoga. Using the hands in various positions to gather in the qi, move the qi, or release the qi is one of the most important aspects of qi gong movements.

The first qi gong exercises you might learn represent the "seasons"—fall, winter, spring, summer, and late summer (there are five seasons here). These exercises look more like a dance than an exercise, with their precise, slow movements.

The word *qi* means vitality, energy, and life force; the word *gong* means practise, cultivate, and refine. The Chinese believe that practising qi gong balances the body and improves physical and mental well-being. These exercises push the life force energy into the various meridian pathways that correspond to organs. It is the same map used in pressure point healing. Qi gong improves oxygen flow and enhances the lymphatic system. Qi gong is similar to tai chi, but allows for greater flexibility in routine. The best way to learn qi gong is through a qualified instructor. You can generally find qi gong classes through the alternative healing community. Check health food stores and other centres that offer classes such as yoga or tai chi. Qi gong is difficult to learn from a book or video.

Deep Breathing

Deep breathing helps to relieve a range of stress-related symptoms, such as anxiety, panic attacks, and irritability. In fact, sighing and yawning are signs that your body isn't getting enough oxygen; the sigh or yawn is your body's way of righting the situation. The following deep breathing techniques are modelled after yogic breathing exercises. Deep breathing calms the nervous system, relaxes the small arteries, and permanently lowers blood pressure.

Abdominal Breathing.
Lie down on a mat or on your bed. Take slow, deep, rhythmic breaths through your nose. When your abdominal cavity is expanded, it means that your lungs have filled completely, which is important. Then, slowly exhale completely, watching your abdomen collapse again. Repeat 6–10 times. Practise this morning and night.

Extended Abdominal Breathing.
Extended abdominal breathing is a variation of the above. When your abdomen expands with air, take three more short inhalations. It's akin to adding those last drops of gas in your tank when your tank is full. Then, after you've exhaled in one long breath, don't inhale yet. Try three more short exhales.

Abdominal Lift.
Stand with feet apart (about shoulder width), bend the knees slightly, bend forward, exhale completely, and brace your hands above the knees. Then lift the abdomen upward while holding your exhalation. Your abdomen should look concave. Stand erect again and inhale just before you feel the urge to gasp. Greer Childers, in her video "Body Flex," demonstrates this technique very well.

Rapid Abdominal Breathing.
This is abdominal breathing done at a fast speed, so it feels as though your inhalations and exhalations are forceful and powerful. Try to do this 25–100 times. Each breath should last only a second or so, compared to the 10–20 seconds involved in regular deep abdominal breathing.

Alternate Nostril Breathing.
Hold one nostril closed, inhaling and exhaling deeply. Then alternate nostrils. This breathing exercise is often done prior to meditation. It is thought to balance the left and right sides of the brain.

Meditation

Meditation simply requires you to stop thinking (about your life, problems, etc.) and just be. To do this, people usually find a relaxing spot, sit quietly, and breathe deeply for a few minutes. Deep breathing isn't always necessary in order to meditate. A number of activities are meditative in the sense that they help you focus and clear your mind. Going for a nature walk, playing golf, listening to music, reading inspiring poetry or prose, gardening, practising qi gong, doing stretching exercises, walking the dog, listening to silence, and listening only to the sound of your own breathing are all forms of meditation.

Meditative Stretching

Stretching improves muscle blood flow, oxygen flow, and digestion. The natural desire to stretch is there for those reasons. The following stretches will help relieve stress and improve tranquility. Many of these are classic yoga postures, too.

- While sitting or standing, raise your arms above your head. Keep the shoulders relaxed and breathe deeply for five seconds. Release and repeat five times.

- Gently raise your shoulders in an exaggerated "shrug." Breathe deeply and hold for 10 seconds. Relax and repeat three times.

- **Lotus.** Sit cross-legged on the floor with spine straight and neck aligned. Focus on your breath, letting it gently fill the diaphragm and the back of the rib cage. On the inhalation, say "so," and on the exhalation, say "hum." Voicing the breath in this manner will keep you focused and relaxed. Continue with "so-hum" until you feel at ease.

- **Child's Pose.** Sit on your heels. Bring your forehead to the floor in front of you. Breathe into the back of the rib cage, feeling the stretch in your spine. Hold as long as it's comfortable.

- **Tree.** Stand tall and find a point across the room at which to focus your gaze. Place the heel of one foot on the opposite inner thigh. Float your arms upward until your palms are touching. Breathe deeply and hold for five seconds. Release and repeat on the other side.

- **Savasana or "Corpse" Pose.** Lie on your back with palms facing upward, feet turned gently outward. Focus on the movement of breath throughout your body.

- **Bow.** Lie on your belly with arms at your sides. Bend your legs at the knees and bring your heels in toward your buttocks. Reach back and take hold of the right, then the left, ankle. Flex your feet if you're having a hard time maintaining this position. Inhale, raising the upper body as far off the floor as possible. Lift your head, completing the arch. Your knees should remain as close together as possible (tying them together might help here). Breathe deeply and hold for 10–15 seconds.

The following postures can also improve digestion:

- **Locust.** Lie on your belly with your arms folded beneath you, palms pressed into your body. Extend both legs until they lift up and off the floor. Keep the toes pointed. Release.

- **Cobra** (Upward Facing Dog). Lie on your belly with your palms down and adjacent to your shoulders. Slowly raise your upper body, lifting all but the lower abdomen toward the ceiling. Breathe deeply. Release.

- **Fish.** Lie on your back. Place your hands under your sitting bones, palms pressed on the floor, feet flexed. Gently roll one, then the other, shoulder inward, shortening the distance between your shoulder blades (your chest will naturally arch upward). Breathe, lengthening your abdominals and rib cage. Release.

- **The Squat.** You simply stand with your feet parallel to your hips and slowly squat down, making sure your weight is forward (rather than reeling backward) and that you don't roll your knees inward. You may need to practise a few times before you can do this comfortably. It's recommended that you "squat" twice a day to aid with constipation.

- **Knee-to-Chest—One Leg.** Lie on your back on the floor. Bend one knee and bring it in to the chest. Then just hug the leg and slowly bring it toward your abdomen. Hold for a count of 10. Relax and repeat with other leg.

- **Knee-to-Chest—Both Legs.** This is the same as the one-leg version, only you will bring both legs to the chest and hug them with both arms, bringing them gently toward your abdomen. Hold them there for a count of 10. Then relax and repeat.

Self-Care

Self-care refers to doing one or two small things just for yourself. Part 1 described the many ways that stress can be manifested physically and emotionally. Part 2 explored the many social causes there are for stress in women—social causes that are completely different than the causes of stress in men. Part 3 presented dozens of suggestions for stress relief—without drugs. This last section gives you a few final self-care suggestions that can help reduce your stress, even if you ignore all of the advice in the rest of Part 3.

Getting Creative

Creativity can dramatically lower stress levels, too. This refers to art in all its forms: words, fine arts, visual arts, healing arts, performing arts, hobbies, or sports. Writing, in the form of a journal, poetry, or correspondence with a friend, is an especially good stress-buster. A new study published in the *Journal of the American Medical Association* found that people suffering from chronic ailments such as asthma or arthritis felt better when they wrote about their health problems.

A few years ago, Oprah Winfrey used her influence to get her viewers to begin writing in a journal or diary on a daily basis; she did this because she recognized that journal writing has a powerful *enabling* effect on those of us who are otherwise without voice or expression. Using her own creativity to enable others, she has "resold" the idea of journal writing in an age where few people take the time to sit down and be still with their thoughts. Oprah has taken journal writing one step further by encouraging people to begin "gratitude journaling," where they think about what, in their lives, they are thankful for and then write about it. Oprah is a firm believer in literacy as well, and by encouraging journal writing, she has given many people the courage to express themselves though writing, people who in the past were afraid to write because of a poor education. For people who don't feel they are "creative" or "artistic," journal writing is an opportunity to express their feelings and passions.

Why is Martha Stewart so successful? Because she offers "creative rescue" for millions through her lifestyle arts. She is essentially the mountain that comes to Mohammed. Martha offers us "good things" that help change our days and routine. When something's called "Martha Stewart Living," it's an invitation to come back to life and feel the small things (which she'll tell you is a good thing), even if it's just to wake up and smell fresh coffee ... *sorbet*. Through her program, magazine, and website, Martha Stewart offers thousands of creative rescues every day, whether it's a beautiful flower arrangement, crafts, or one of the hundreds of small things that take hours to make.

Do What You Loved as a Child

Children are naturally filled with creativity and passion; they're so enamoured with life that they don't want to sleep and can barely wait to start each day. Believe it or not, you were like that once, too. Make a list of activities, foods, or places you enjoyed as a child and re-enact the memory today. Take a ride on a roller coaster; have some candy floss; finger paint; play in the snow; eat dinner backwards, with dessert first; play with some toys. One creativity expert refers to this as "Rekindlegarten." The feelings we had as children when we did these kinds of things can be brought back, and those feelings can jump start a childlike quality that can keep us feeling young, creative, and passionate.

That childlike feeling has a lot to do with fearlessness. When we try something new, we re-create the wonder we felt as children when we tried something for the first time. There are lots of things that all of us can try for the first time! Here are a few suggestions, listed from the more conservative to the wild:

- Try a new restaurant.
- Take in a tourist attraction in your own city that you've never been to.
- Go to a sports event you've never attended before.
- Take an architecture tour of your city, and look at buildings and shapes in a new way.
- Throw a party just like that.
- Take dancing lessons.
- Go on a nature adventure (e.g., whitewater rafting).
- Dress up in formal wear and go to the beach.
- Go for a helicopter ride.

You get the idea! The point is, try something totally new and "unlike" you.

Try Out Feng Shui

Our surroundings have a lot to do with how we feel. One of the energy drains discussed in Chapter 8 was unattractive surroundings. If you are interested in making your surroundings more attractive and hence more of a haven for yourself, you might be interested in investigating *feng shui* (pronounced "fung shway"). Feng shui is the ancient practice of creating energy and harmony through environmental surroundings (landscaping, interior design, architecture). People tend to think of feng shui as something that can bring them wealth (as in money corners) or romance (as in hanging certain items over the bed), but this is not what authentic feng shui consultants have in mind. Harmony has many elements to it, and where you live, how you live, and a host of other geographic particulars all affect how you might best arrange your environment. Feng shui consultants will assess the following:

- **Entrances.** How is your entrance lit? What do you have at your entrance (hanging flowers, chimes, or a stack of old newspapers)?
- **Grounds.** What kinds or colours of flowers are around your home; are there rocks or sculptures on the grounds of your home?
- **Specific areas** (your work space/home office, "chef station" or kitchen, bedroom, bathroom, and so on). The placement of mirrors, pictures, plants, lamps, candles, rugs, furniture, bed, or even aquariums is significant. For example, round or octagonal mirrors are powerful and should be positioned to advantage.

In general, the feng shui consultant tries to optimize the grounds surrounding your space through curvilinear and rectangular visual contours or edges, wildlife, landscaping/vegetation, and aquatic habitat, and to minimize things that interfere with harmony, such as signage, power lines, and so forth. Inside the home, plants, colours, lighting, and the positioning of furniture to maximize views of natural scenery are important. Feng shui is said to reduce stress, blood pressure, and adrenaline levels. A good way to begin is with a book on feng shui. There are dozens of these!

Avoid Loneliness

Loneliness is stressful; solitude is not. Loneliness comes from a lack of truly intimate relationships with friends or family members; intimacy, in this case, refers to sharing deep feelings, fears, and so on with someone. This is how we unburden ourselves and relieve stress. Feeling as though we belong somewhere or are part of a community can also alleviate loneliness.

The large body of work that looks at causes of depression in women shows us that people suffer most when they feel that they've lost their connection with the world around them. The feeling of being "plugged in" to our community and network of friends and colleagues brings us increased zest, well-being, and motivation. Connection increases our sense of self-worth, as well as a desire to make more connections. The flip side of wanting to connect with someone is fearing that if we open up too much we'll become vulnerable. Vulnerability can, of course, lead to our being taken advantage of. Most people, at some time or another, have allowed less than savoury characters into their lives when they were vulnerable or open. A lot of us may stray into relationships with people who take terrible advantage of our feelings and openness. The problem with vulnerability is that it cannot be halfway. There is simply no way around this risk. This is why many of us learn to shut down. And when we shut down, passion is repressed, which can predispose us to depression or numbness. Here are steps you can take to establish supportive relationships in your life:

Find a Social Group That Suits You.

You can find a compatible group by looking into gourmet cooking clubs, art classes, and so on. Focus on an activity that you're really drawn to, and chances are, you'll meet like-minded souls with whom you can form quality friendships.

Have a Couple of Nice Dinner Parties Each Year.

This is a way to create more intimate friendships with people who, unless an effort is made, will remain only acquaintances or casual friends.

Get Involved in Your Community.

Stories from New York after September 11, 2001, show how valuable community support can be. Whether it's a "not in my backyard" lobby or a community street sale, get out and meet your neighbours. Responding to community-based programs, ranging from crafts groups to yoga classes, is the way to find supportive friends. In fact, community outreach workers deliberately use the arts, crafts, fitness, computer classes, and so on to attract people within the community who could benefit from support. What often takes place in community-based programs is a great deal of talking and sharing during, prior to, or after the activity. These are places where you make friends, find someone you can talk to, and, most importantly, find that you're not alone.

Volunteer.
Volunteering for causes dear to your heart is a great way to meet people and feel needed. Meals On Wheels, eldercare facilities, street youth programs, and so forth all attract wonderful souls with whom you may find friendship and comfort.

Get a Dog.
Dogs need to be walked, which means you'll meet other people walking their dogs. And dog owners tend to gravitate toward other dog owners. Dog walking is a great jumping-off point for meeting people. Aside from that, many studies point to the health effects of pet ownership, including lower blood pressure and a lower incidence of heart disease. (Positive health effects can be seen with any pet, including cats!!)

Pamper Yourself

Taking care of yourself means being good to yourself. Give yourself some TLC. You'll find this goes a long way in battling daily stresses. Here are some suggestions:

Set Aside "Comfort Time" for Yourself.
You should give yourself comfort time at least once a week. Make it a ritual. It can be having coffee with your morning paper, going for a scenic stroll, window shopping in a favourite neighbourhood, taking a long bath, going to an open market (these are often on the weekends), or having breakfast in bed once a week. All these are feel-good activities that will make you feel energized and loved.

Have a Very Long Shower Each Morning.
Treat yourself to a shower massage and take time to massage every part of your body. Buy energizing shower gels or shower "toys" to use each day.

Have a Steam Bath.
Run the shower and sit in your bathroom on a mat and just enjoy the steam.
Have a luxurious bubble bath. Using aromatherapy to augment your bath can work wonders for relieving stress (see Table 10.1). For a spa-style bath, use mud products, dried milk powder for a milk bath, or mineral salts for aching muscles. The bath ritual can be enhanced with candlelight, music, and moisturizing oils or lotions applied after the bath.

Take a Bed-Rest Day.

Change the linens, fluff up your pillows, lay in a supply of good reading material, prepare a tray of favourite snacks, wine, coffee, tea, etc., and go to bed. Take the day as a "sick day" and rejuvenate.

Plan a "Spa Day."

You can take this as a sick day if you like. Start your day in the bath (see above). Then, go outside for a nice long walk. Come back inside and take an invigorating shower, scrubbing your body with a loofah scrubber or rough washcloth. Then, wash your hair and put in a deep conditioning treatment. Leave shower, stay in bathroom, and begin to smooth the calluses on your feet. Start another bath with essential oils. Cleanse your face well and apply your favourite facial mask. Light candles and soak, with a cool washcloth over your eyes. Then, get back in the shower, rinse off the mask, and remoisturize your body. Wrap yourself in a towel and take a nap. (You may want to arrange in advance for a massage therapist to visit you at this point!) After your nap, make a nice "smoothie" with your favourite fruits. And then order in from your favourite restaurant to top off the day. Go to bed early with a book or magazine and a bed tray of snacks or leftovers!

Enjoy Your Food

The French have a saying that's derived from the lyric of an old French torch song: *Regret nothing—in matters of love and food.* Scientists who've been puzzling over why the French have such low rates of heart disease in spite of their diet of heavy cream sauces (their good health is known as the "French Paradox") have found that the answer is passion. The French are passionate about their food and really enjoy it. They never think of food as sinful; instead, they simply think of it as tasty. To the French, food is a work of art, meant to be enjoyed. To the North American, food is "fattening" and "forbidden." North Americans tend to think about food as either fuel or poison; they fear the effect the food will have on their bodies. In France, good food feeds the *soul,* not the body. (Apparently, General de Gaulle used to say, "It's difficult to govern a country that has 500 varieties of cheese.") In France, people mock the idea of "food police" counting every gram of fat. What is also mocked is the way North Americans eat: everywhere and anywhere is a dining room. We eat in our cars, while walking on the street, and at our desks when we work. In France, people eat in restaurants or at dinner tables. The French consider the North American pattern of eating to be nomadic eating, or vagabond feeding and grazing. There is also a huge distinction between quantity and quality of food. In North America, we are taught that large portions are good—even if the food is mediocre and of poor quality. In France, the quality and taste of the food are the most important factors: when taste is there and the quality of the food is high, the diner is satisfied—quantity or portion size is not important. When food is enjoyed, endorphins are secreted, relieving stress. One of the most well-known comfort foods, chocolate, has been found to have this effect.

Cry More, Laugh More, and Learn to Forgive

Stress relief comes from the release of stress hormones. One of the best ways to do this is to have a good cry. Human tears contain high levels of stress hormone, which is one reason why people who cry tend to have less stress than those who don't cry. A dramatic movie can induce tears, hence the term "tear-jerker." These movies serve important purposes if you feel you need a good cry.

Laughter is another way to reduce stress because it makes us feel good, boosting endorphin levels in our body. Laughter also causes deep muscle relaxation (which is why you can sometimes lose bladder control). Our blood pressure drops, while the T-cells in our immune system increase. Incorporating humour into your life can be fun, too. Look for humorous books, magazines, or other material, and keep them handy. Get yourself onto a humour listserv. Rent funny videos; watch comedy networks; and use laughter to diffuse stress at the office and at home. Laughter bonds people and also attracts people to you. Teachers, doctors, or salespeople who generate laughter have more loyal students, more compliant patients, and higher sales.

The final great stress-reliever is forgiveness. When you have unresolved conflict with someone or you're nursing a grudge, the emotional weight you carry increases blood pressure, stress hormones, heart rate, perspiration, and muscle tenseness. Forgiveness doesn't mean excusing bad behaviour, but it does mean that you are prepared to move forward and let go of your bitterness toward that person. Forgiveness is healthier for you, and chances are, the person with whom you are in conflict would either welcome your forgiveness or, if also nursing a grudge, would, deep down, want to forgive you, too.

Forgiveness is about saying the "Serenity Prayer" (accepting the things you cannot change; changing the things you can). You can't change the fact that the conflict occurred, but you can change your current response to that conflict.

Bibliography

"Addicted to the Urge to Splurge: Tis the Season for All to Spend, but So-Called Shopaholics Find It Hard to Say No at the Best of Times." *Maclean's* (Toronto edition) 108, no. 50 (December 11, 1995): 58–59.

Agin, Beth. "Treating Myself to a Weekend of Simple Pleasure." Focus on Forty. Retrieved from www. focusonforty.com (2001).

"Alcohol and Women." Retrieved September 25, 2001 from www.oprah.com.

"All about You: De-stress [readership survey results]." *Flare* 20, no. 8 (August 1998): 82–83. Illustrations.

"All Work and No Play." *Canada and the World Backgrounder* 62, no. 5 (March 1997): 22–25.

Allardice, Pamela. *Essential Oils: The Fragrant Art of Aromatherapy.* Vancouver: Raincoast Books, 1999.

"Allergies, Common Colds Often Share Symptoms but Need Different Medications." retrieved from www.cnn.com (April 18, 2000).

Anderson, Carol M., Susan Stewart with Sona Dimidjian. *Flying Solo.* New York: W. Norton & Company, 1994.

Andre, Pierre, and Bernard Jean. "Mental Health and Relocation: Towards a Synthesis." *Environments* 22, no. 1 (1993): 37–53. Graphics; bibliography.

"Antidepressants' Impact Mainly from Boost of Getting Treated, Study Suggests." Associated Press, July 20, 1998.

"Anxiety Disorders." Retrieved from National Institute of Mental Health, National Institutes of Health, Bethesda, MD 20892, 1994 (September 25, 2001).

Apple, Alvin. "Gender Equality in Business: We've Come a Long Way, but We Still Have a Long Way to Go." Retrieved from www. leatherspinsters.com/genderequality.html (July 2001).

"Aromatherapy for Stress Relief." Concerning Women. Retrieved from http://www. concerningwomen.com/wl_article6.html (September 25, 2001).

Baker, Sandy. "The Number One Way to Eliminate Daily Stress. *The National Public Account,* no. 10 (December 2000): 13.

"The Balancing Act: Can We Find Time for Work and Family?" *Today's Parent* 11, no. 2 (April 1994): 42–46.

Ballweg, Rachel. "7 Simple Ways to Reduce Stress." *Better Homes and Gardens* 78, no. 1 (January 2000): 62.

Banda Purvis, Sarah. "Lessons Learned: The Myth of Workplace Equity." *Feminista!* 3, no. 2 (June 1999), www.feminista.com/v3n2/ purvis.html.

Bass, Frederic, and Lynn Wilson. "Kicking the Nicotine Habit." *Medical Post* 34, no. 41 (December 1, 1998): Q1–Q7. Illustrations; graphs.

"Beating the Cash Crunch (Money Makeovers)." *Flare* 17, no. 1 (January, 1995): 36–37.

Beaudet, Marie P., and Claudio Perez. "The Health of Lone Mothers [1994–1997 data; first part of full text]." *Health Reports* 11, no. 2 (Fall 1999): 21–32.

Beers, David. "Take This Overtime and Shove It." Retrieved from www.rabble.ca/news_full_story. shtml?x=1403 (June 21, 2001).

———. "Terminally Addicted." Retrieved from www.rabble.ca/news_full_story.shtml?x=211 (May 14, 2001).

Ben-Ari, Elia T. "Walking the Tightrope between Work and Family." *BioScience* 50, no. 5 (May 2000): 472.

Bennetts, Leslie. "e-Stress." *FamilyPC* 7, no. 6 (June 200): 93.

Bertolis, Dimitra, and Judi Lewis. "Questions about the Glass Ceiling Situation." Retrieved from www.theglassceiling.com/glass/ ww6_32.htm (September 25, 2001).

Björk, Malin. "Take 3 Minutes to Read These Figures—Angry." Retrieved from www.worldwoman.net/politics/ tangry36200122576.html (March 6, 2001).

Block, Jennifer. "Work Notes: Laugh Lines." *Ms. Magazine,* June/July 2000.

Blonz, Ed. "Grandma's Penicillin." *Better Homes and Gardens,* October 1998.

Boll, Rosemarie. "The Mathematics of Divorce." *Law Now* 20, no. 6 (June/July 1996): 36.

Borah, Kitty, and Stacy Hutchinson. "The Shell Poll 'Mars and Venus' Agree Equality of the Sexes Needs to Go Further." Retrieved from www.theglassceiling.com/glass/shell.htm (February 23, 2000).

Boulware, Carole. "Is My Anxiety Normal, Part I." retrieved from www.therapyinla.com. (June 1999)

Bourette, Susan. "New Wave Women: For Women, the Road to the Top Is Fraught with Twists, Turns and Potholes That Men Rarely Notice." *CMA Management* 73, no. 3 (April 1999): 14–17.

Bowen, Jon. "Fisticuffs in the Cube: Stressed-Out Office Workers Are Succumbing to 'Desk Rage.'" Retrieved from www.salon.com (September 7, 1999).

Bower, Peter J., et al. "Manual Therapy: Hands-on Healing." *Patient Care* 31, no. 20 (December, 15, 1997): 69.

"Breaking the Silence [accounts of women who have left abusive situations]." *Windspeaker* 11, no. 17 (November 8/21, 1993): 12–16.

Brennan, Moira. "Work Notes." *Ms. Magazine,* December 1999/January 2000.

Brook, Paula. "Superwoman Goes Home: I Had It All. I'd Also Had Enough." *Saturday Night* 111, no. 5 (June 1996): 30–38.

Cardwell, Mark. "Career Plus Family Equals High Blood Pressure for Women: Canadian Study Focused on Educated Women." *Medical Post* 35, no. 16 (April 27, 1999): 12.

Carelse, Michele. "How to Stop Smoking." Retrieved from www.allthatwomenwant.com/ smoking.html (September 25, 2001).

Carey, Elaine. "Hunger a Fear for 3 Million Canadians." *Toronto Star,* August 16, 2001.

Carlson, Betty Clark. "Managing Time for Personal Effectiveness: Achieving Goals with Less Stress." *ISMA-USA Newsletter* 1, no. 1 (Spring 1999).

Carlson, John G. "Relax Your Way to Stress Management." International Stress Management Association. Retrieved from ISMA library www.isma.org.uk (June 2000).

Carr, Martha, and Heather Davis. "Gender Differences in Arithmetic Strategy Use: A Function of Skill and Preference." *Contemporary Educational Psychology* 26 (2001): 330–347.

Carrier, Patricia J., and Lorraine Davies. "The Importance of Power Relations for the Division of Household Labour." *Canadian Journal of Sociology* 24, no. 1 (Winter 99): 35–51.

Carter, Peter. "The Fixers: When You See a Canadian Workplace Getting Better, Healthier, Friendlier, More Community-Minded, Chances Are a Woman Got Things Moving." *Chatelaine* 73, no. 11 (November 2000): 78–87. Illustrations.

Cass, Hyla. *St. John's Wort: Nature's Blues Buster.* New York: Avery Publishing Group, 1998.

Chatterji, Shoma. "When the Wife Earns More." Retrieved from www.moxiemag.com/moxie/ articles/work/earnsmore.html (August 5, 2000).

Chaudhry, Lakshmi. "Married to the Visa." *Ms. Magazine.* Retrieved from www.msmagazine.com. (April 18, 2001)

Cheung, Cindy. "Lots of Barriers out There and in There." Retrieved from www.theglassceiling.com/glass/ww7_46.htm (September 25, 2001).

Chisholm, Patricia. "The Mother Load: Superwoman Is Burned Out. Should Mom Stay Home?" *Maclean's* (Toronto edition) 112, no. 9 (March 1, 1999): 46.

Christensen, Carole-P., and Morton Weinfeld. "The Black Family in Canada: A Preliminary Exploration of Family Patterns and Inequality." *Canadian Ethnic Studies* 25, no. 3 (1993): 26–44.

Christmas Derrick, Rachel. "Less Stress on the Job." *Essence* 30, no. 11 (March 2000): 44.

Cicala, Roger S. *The Heart Disease Sourcebook.* Los Angeles: Lowell House, 1998.

Clarke, Bill. "Action Figures." *Diabetes Dialogue* 43, no. 3 (Fall 1996).

Clarke, Robyn D., "Serenity Now." *Black Enterprise* 30, no. 6 (January 2000): 115.

Cohen, Bruce. "CPP Credit System Can Work against Divorced Couples: Retirement Expert Discovers Drop-Out Periods Wipe Out Ex-Wife's Benefits." *Financial Post* (*National Post*) April 30, 1999, D4.

Cohen, May. "Cracking the Glass Ceiling" *Canadian Medical Association Journal* 157, no. 12 (December 15, 1997): 1713–1714.

Collins, Rosemary. "Flex Appeal: Flexible Work Arrangements Are Increasingly Popular with Bank Employees." *Canadian Banker* 104, no. 3 (May/June 1997): 12–16.

"Combat Job Stress: Does Work Make You Sick?" Retrieved from www.convoke.com/markjr/cjstress.html (February 12, 1999).

"Coming to Terms with Grief after a Longtime Partner Dies." *New York Times* (national edition), June 13, 1999, 10.

"Complications of the Common Cold." Retrieved from www.commoncold.org (October 18, 2001).

"Compressed Work Week Stressful for Women, Says Stats Can." Canadian Press newswire, January 7, 1997.

"Coping with Addiction." Retrieved from www.oprah.com (September 25, 2001).

"Coping with stress: Canadians Look for New Ways to Reduce Pressures That Threaten Their Careers, Families and Even Health." *Maclean's* (Toronto edition) 109, no. 2 (January 8, 1996): 32–36. Photograph.

Cornelius, Coleman. "Brave New Mom." *Fit Pregnancy,* February/March 2000, www.fitpregnancy.com.

Cornell, Camilla. "The Toughest Job of All: You're Leaving the Nest and Returning to Work. Here's How to Ease the Emotional Adjustment." *Today's Parent* 15, no. 2 (March 1998): 48–54.

Costin, Carolyn. *The Eating Disorder Sourcebook.* Los Angeles: Lowell House/Chicago: Contemporary Books, 1996.

Cotton, Paul. "Environmental Estrogenic Agents Area of Concern." *Journal of the American Medical Association* 271 (9 February 1994): 414, 416.

Cox, Meg. "Zero Balance." *Ms. Magazine,* February/March 2001.

Crawford, Trish. "Long-Term Marriages Are Disintegrating Like Never Before." Canadian Press newswire, May 28, 2001.

"Creating a Love That Will Last." One-day workshop presented by Louise Dorfman and David Rubinstein, Couple Enrichment Inc., October 28, 2001.

Crittenden, Danielle. "The Mother of All Problems: Every Woman Knows What Her Child Needs Most Is Her." *Saturday Night* 111, no. 3 (April 1996): 44–50.

Cummings, Melanie. "Women Who Do Too Much (or Feel Guilty If They Don't)." *Herizons* 11, no. 4 (Fall 1997): 25–26. Illustration.

Curtis, Patricia. "Stress-Free Zone." *Redbook* 194, no. 6 (June 2000): 157.

Dadd, Debra Lynn. *The Nontoxic Home and Office*. Los Angeles: Jeremy P. Tarcher, 1992.

Datao, Robert. "The Law of Stress." International Stress Management Association. Retrieved from www.datodevelopment.com (June 2000).

Davies, Lorraine, and Donna D. McAlpine. "The Significance of Family, Work, and Power Relations for Mothers' Mental Health [2nd part of full text]." *Canadian Journal of Sociology* 23, no. 4 (Fall 1998): 369–387. Tables; bibliography.

Davis, Martha, Elizabeth Robbins Eshelman, and Matthew McKay. *The Relaxation and Stress Reduction Workbook*. Oakland, CA: New Harbinger, 1995.

Delanet, Kathy, and Marie R. Squillace. *Living with Heart Disease*. Los Angeles: Lowell House, 1998.

"Depression & Drugs: Women Suffer Depression at More Than Twice the Rate of Men." *Flare* 18, no. 4 (April 1996): 85–86.

"Divorce and Single Parenthood." *MsMoney*. Retrieved from www.msmoney.com/mm/planning/divorce/divorce_intro.htm (September 10, 2001).

"Divorce and Your Mental Health." *Health News* 17, no. 3 (June/July 1999): 5.

"Divorce Rate Rises in 1998 for the First Time in Four Years, Says StatsCan." Canadian Press newswire, September 28, 2000.

"Divorce Report a Recipe for Chaos [Joint Committee on Child Custody and Access final report]." *Herizons* 12, no. 4 (Winter 1999): 11–12. Illustrations.

"Divorced People More Likely to Seek Psychiatric Help Than Married Ones." *Health News* 17, no. 1 (February/March 1999): 11.

Dobkind, Doris. "Ten Delightful Ways to Get a Little Extra Cash." Retrieved from www.allthatwomenwant.com/extracash.htm (2000).

Douglas, Ann. *Sanity Savers: The Canadian Working Woman's Guide to (Almost) Having It All*. Toronto: McGraw-Hill Ryerson, 1999.

Douglas, Susan, and Meredith Michaels. "Mommy Wars." *Ms. Magazine*, February/March 2000.

Dreher, Henry, and Domar, Alice D. *Healing Mind, Healthy Woman*. New York: Henry Holt and Co., 1996.

"Emotional Abusers." Retrieved from Heartless Bitches International. www.heartlessbitches.com/rants/emotional_abuse.shtml (September 25, 2001).

"Employment Challenges Facing Women" [excerpt from 1999 annual report]. *Worklife Report* 12, no. 3 (2000): 10–11.

"Energy Drains." Retrieved from www.oprah.com (September 25, 2001).

Engel, June V. "Beyond Vitamins: Phytochemicals to Help Fight Disease." *Health News* 14 (June 1996).

Enzo, Iammetteo. "The Alexander Technique: Improving the Balance." *Performing Arts and Entertainment in Canada* 30, no. 3 (Fall 1996): 37.

Evans, Julie A. "Stop Back Pain Instantly!" *Prevention* 51, no. 7 (July 1999): 128.

"Family-Friendly Workplaces." *Canadian Business Review* 21, no. 2 (Summer 1994): 44. Graphic.

Faret, Liv. "A Few Points about the Glass Ceiling." Retrieved from www.theglassceiling.com/glass/ww1_35.htm (September 25, 2001).

———. "The Film Industry and the Glass Ceiling" Retrieved from www.theglassceiling.com/glass/glass3.htm (September 25, 2001).

"Fatigue Tops List of Women's Health Worries" [study by Toronto Hospital's Women's Health Program]. Canadian Press newswire, June 20, 1996.

"A Field Guide to Stress: A Conversation with Kenneth R. Pelletier, Ph.D." *Selfcare Archives,* December 15, 1997.

"Forgiving Others." Retrieved from www.oprah.com (September 25, 2001).

Fransen, Jenny, and I. Jon Russell. *The Fibromyalgia Help Book*. Smith House Press, 1996.

Fredman, Catherine. "How to Give a Back Rub." *Ladies Home Journal* 117, no. 4 (April 2000): 66.

Friedan, Betty. *The Feminine Mystique*. First edition. New York: W.W. Norton, 1963.

Fugh-Berman, Adriane. *Alternative Medicine: What Works*. Tucson, AZ: Odonian Press, 1996.

Galarneau, Diane, and Louise Earl. "Women's Earnings, Men's Earnings." *Perspectives on Labour and Income* (Statscan) 11, no. 4 (Winter 1999): 20–26.

"Get Herbal Relief." *Prevention* 51, no. 7 (July 1999): 128.

"Getting to the Roots of a Vegetarian Diet." Vegetarian Resource Group, Baltimore, MD, 1997.

Gillespie, Marcia Ann. "Mothering Our Mothers." *Ms. Magazine*, June/July 2001.

"Going over the Edge: For Most People, the Family Is a Place of Safety, Nurturing and Positive Values. For Others, Violence Turns Family Life into a Nightmare." *Canada and the World Backgrounder* 62, no. 5 (March 1997): 26–27.

Goulston, Mark. "Yes, There's Life (and Even Love) after Divorce." *Business Woman* 84, no. 4 (Summer 2000): 13.

Govier, Katherine. "Women and Money." *Toronto Life* 32, no. 2 (February 98): 68–72.

Gower, Dave. "Retirement Patterns of Working Couples." *Perspectives on Labour and Income* (Statscan) 10, no. 3 (Fall 1998): 27–30. Tables; bibliography.

Greenberg, Brigitte. "Stress Hormone Linked to High-Fat Snacking in Women." Associated Press newswire, April 4, 1998.

Grout, Pam. "Tune Out Stress." *Ingram's* 21, no. 4 (April 1995): 78.

Gunawant, Deepika, and Gopi Warrier. *Ayurveda: The Ancient Indian Healing Tradition*. Rockport, MA: New Element Books, 1997.

Haas, Elson M. "Anti-Stress Nutritional Program." *HealthWorld Online*. Retrieved from www.healthy.net (June 2000).

Hadley, Karen. "Gender and Restructuring." *Atlantis* 23, no. 2 (Spring 1999).

Hamilton, Tim, and Satish Sharma. "Family Violence and Anti-Oppressive Family Counseling." *Peace Research* 29, no. 1 (February 1997): 25–40.

Harvey, Steve, and Julia Scott. "Men's and Women's Investment Habits: Investors Seem to Be as Risk Adverse as Ever." *Canadian Investment Review* 10, no. 2 (Summer 97): 17–19.

"Headaches." Women's Health Interactive. Retrieved from www.whi.com (October 18, 2001).

Helgerson, Kristine. "'Honey, There's Somebody Else.' When One Spouse Strays, a Lot More Than Trust Is Lost." *Chatelaine* 72, no. 7 (July 1999): 24f–24j.

Hendler, Saul Sheldon. *The Doctors' Vitamin and Mineral Encyclopedia*. New York: Fireside Books, 1990.

Herring, Jeff. "Bring Back Passion to Your Everyday Life." Knight Ridder/Tribune News Service, February 21, 2000, pK0535.

———. "Use These 10 Tips to Manage Stress." Knight Ridder/Tribune News Service, January 31, 2000, pK0817.

———. "You Can Manage Stress with HALTS." Knight-Ridder/Tribune News Service, May 22, 2000, pK1632.

Hite, Shere. *Sex and Business*. Toronto: Prentice Hall Canada, 2000.

Ho, Marian. "Learning Your ABCs, Part Two." *Diabetes Dialogue* 43, No. 3 (Fall 1996).

Hoffman, David L. "Herbal Remedies and Stress Management." *HealthWorld Online*. Retrieved from www.healthy.net (June 2000).

———. "The Nervous System and Herbal Remedies." *HealthWorld Online.* Retrieved from www.healthy.net (June 2000).

Holcomb, Betty. "Friendly for Whose Family." *Ms. Magazine,* April/May 2000.

Hopson, Emma, and Judi Light Hopson. *Burnout to Balance: EMS Stress.* New York: Simon & Schuster/Brady Books, 2000.

"Hostility and Heart Risk." *Reuters Health Summary,* April 22, 1997.

House, Michelle. "Gender Wage Gap in Nonprofit Sector." *Nervygirl.* Retrieved from www.nervygirlzine.com/nervy/July_2001/news.html#one (July/Aug 2001).

"How Forgiving Helps You." *Redbook* 194, no. 3 (March 2000): 36.

Hunt, Paula. "Touch Up." *Vegetarian Times,* November 1999, 96.

"Influenza." National Foundation for Infectious Diseases. Retrieved from www.nfid.org (October 21, 2001).

"Irritable Bowel Syndrome Linked to Emotional Abuse." *Tufts University Health & Nutrition Letter* 18, no. 2 (April 2000): 3.

"Is Your Lifestyle Ruining Your Health." Retrieved from www.oprah.com (September 25, 2001).

"It's a Jungle Out There! Why Stress in the 1990s Is a Whole Different Animal." *Canadian Occupational Safety* 32, no. 4 (July/August 1994): 14–17.

Jacobsen, Sharon. "Surviving Life after Divorce." Retrieved from www.allthatwomenwant.com/afterdivorce.htm (September 25, 2001).

Jamieson, John, Karen Flood, and Norman Lavoie. "Physical Fitness and Heart Rate Recovery from Stress." *Canadian Journal of Behavioural Science* 26, no. 4 (October 1994): 566–577.

"Jane's Addiction (Women and Addiction)." *Flare* 18, no. 8 (August 1996): 68–72.

Jarboe, Edel. "Stress Management and Your Quality of Life." Retrieved from www.selfhelpforher.com/health13.htm (September 25, 2001).

Jensen-Phyllis-M. "A History of Women and Smoking." *Canadian Woman Studies* 14, no. 3 (Summer 1994): 29–32. Photograph; bibliography.

Jetter, Alexis. "Uppity Women: Wynona Ward." *Ms. Magazine,* February/March 2000.

"Job Sharing Gives Women Best of Both Worlds." Canadian Press newswire, June 10, 1997.

"Job-Home Conflicts Recipe for 'Supermom Disease.'" Canadian Press newswire, March 22, 1995.

Joffe, Russell, and Anthony Levitt. *Conquering Depression.* Hamilton: Empowering Press, 1998.

Johnson, Catherine. *When to Say Goodbye to Your Therapist.* New York: Simon and Schuster, 1988.

Johnson, Lois Joy. "You Look Divine: Stress Management Techniques." *Ladies Home Journal* 117, no. 1 (January 2000): 92.

Johnson, Susan. "Sexual Harassment—Making It Through." *Vicit Vim Virtus.* Retrieved from www.gojobrights.com/Articles/19991001vol5mecca.html (November 1999).

Joplin, Janice. "The Therapeutic Benefits of Expressive Writing." *The Academy of Management Executive* 14, no. 2 (May 2000): 124.

"Just Say No: Here's How to Stop Trying to Please Everyone." *Flare* 15, no. 8 (August 1993): 56, 58.

Kalbfleisch, Robin. "Eldercare Major Source of Stress for Working Women." *Canadian Healthcare Manager* 6, no. 6 (October/November 1999): 11.

Kaptchuk, Ted, and Micheal Croucher. *The Healing Arts: A Journal through the Faces of Medicine.* London: British Broadcasting Corporation, 1986.

Kaslof, Leslie J. "Natural Substances Offer New Hope for Stress Relief." *HealthWorld Online.* Retrieved from www.healthy.net (June 2000).

Keating, Daniel P. "What Everyone Should Know about Middle Age." *Canadian Speeches* 6, no. 10 (February 1993): 42–46.

Keenan, Tia R. "Women's Work: Child Care Worker." *Ms. Magazine,* June 1999.

"Keeping Women in Line." News segment. Produced by ABCNews *20/20,* originally aired July 21, 1995, and re-aired June 21, 1996.

Keyishian, Amy. "Calming Rituals for Rotten Days." *Cosmopolitan* 228, no. 2 (February 2000): 152.

"Kicking the Habit." Retrieved from www.abc.com (September 25, 2001).

"Kicking the Habit: At last, a Treatment That Combats Craving." *Scientific American.* Retrieved from www.sciam.com (January 2, 2000).

"Kids, Careers and the Day Care Debate." *Maclean's* (Toronto edition) 106, no. 22 (May 31, 1993): 36–40.

Kishi, Misa. "Impact of Pesticides on Health in Developing Countries: Research, Policy and Actions." Paper presented at the World Conference on Breast Cancer, July 13–17, 1997, Kingston, Ontario.

Kock, Henry. "Restoring Natural Vegetation as Part of the Farm." *Gardening without Chemicals '91* (Canadian Organic Growers, Toronto Chapter), April 6, 1991.

Kohl, Lisa, et al. "One Woman vs. Working Woman Magazine." *Shatter the Glass Ceiling.* Retrieved from www.theglassceiling.com/glass/glass6.htm (May 14, 1998).

Kong, Dolores. "Women Investors Look to the Future." *Financial Post* (*National Post*), December 2, 2000, E6.

Kotulak, Ronald. "Researchers: Lack of Sleep May Cause Aging, Stress, Flab." *Chicago Tribune,* April 5, 1998.

Kuczmarski R.J, et al. "Increasing Prevalence of Overweight among U.S. Adults: The National Health and Nutrition Examination Surveys, 1960 to 1991. *Journal of the American Medical Association* 272 (1994): 205–211.

Kushi, Mishio. *The Cancer Prevention Guide.* New York: St. Martin's Press, 1993.

Lad, Dr. Vasant. Ayurveda: The Science of Self-Healing. Santa Fe: Lotus Press: 1984.

Lang, Amanda. "When Work Rules: If You Take the Office Everywhere, You May Be One of the New Workaholics." *Flare* 19, no. 11 (November 1997): 106–110. Illustration.

Lark, Susan. *Chronic Fatigue and Tiredness.* Los Altos, CA: Westchester Publishing Co., 1993.

Laver, Ross. "Pensions and Divorce: A Recent Court Ruling in Ottawa Highlights One of the Hidden Costs of Marriage Breakdown [Ted and Marlene Best case]." (Toronto edition) 111, no. 3 (January 19, 1998): 48.

Lemay, Tracy. "Sisters, You'd Better Start Saving for Yourselves: Live Longer, Spend More." *Financial Post* (*National Post*), December 16, 2000, C4.

Lemonick, Michael D. "Eat Your Heart Out." *Time,* July 19, 1999.

Lerner, Harriet Goldhor. *The Dance of Anger.* New York: HarperCollins, 1997.

Levin, Linda. "When Domestic Violence Shows Up at Work." *National Business Woman* 76, no. 1 (Spring 1995): 117.

Lewis, Judi. "The 'good ole boy' syndrome strikes again." *Shatter the Glass Ceiling.* Retrieved from www.theglassceiling.com/glass/ww12_goo.htm (September 3, 2000).

———. "The Academic Glass Ceiling." *Shatter the Glass Ceiling.* Retrieved online from www.theglassceiling.com/glass/ww1_33.htm (June 1997).

Linden, Wolfgang, et al. "Recommendations on Stress Management" [lifestyle modifications to

prevent and control hypertension supplement].
Canadian Medical Association Journal 160, no. 9
(May 4, 1999): S46–S49.

Lippert Gray. "Carol Get a Life." Financial
Executives Institute, 2000. Article A62599863.

"Listen to the Kids: Not Surprisingly, the Broken
Families, the Cultural Conflicts ... Are Taking
Their Toll on Kids, but the News Isn't All Bad."
Canada and the World Backgrounder 62, no. 5
(March 1997): 20–21.

Liu, Lynda, "A Good Cry." *Teen Magazine* 44, no.
6 (June 2000): 38.

Lloyd, Joan "Been Home Raising a Family? Don't
Be Embarrassed about It!" *All That Women Want.*
Retrieved from www.allthatwomenwant.
com/returningtowork.htm (September 25, 2001).

Lock, Craig. "The Facts of Life—Money
Management for Women" *All That Women Want.*
Retrieved from www.allthatwomenwant.com/
moneymanagement.htm (September 25, 2001).

MacPhail, Fiona. "A Feminist Economics
Perspective on Recent Trends in Inequity in
Canada." *Atlantis* 23, no. 2 (Spring 1999).

"Making Work Work for Parents" [highlights of
the Canadian National Child Care Study].
Today's Parent 11, no. 4 (June/July 1994): 17.

Mallet, Gina. "Elaine Calder [Coping with Stress
& Strain on the Job]." *Financial Post Magazine,*
April 1999, 32.

———. "Kimberly Glasco [Coping with Stress &
Strain on the Job]." *Financial Post Magazine,*
April 1999, 28. Illustrations.

———. "Spotlight on Success: The Canadian
Woman Entrepreneur of the Year Awards."
Financial Post Magazine, December 1997, 82–91.

Malone, Catherine. "Equity and Me: My Life as
an Employment Equity Practitioner." *Atlantis* 23,
no. 2 (Spring 1999).

Manji, Irshad. "The Breakthrough Syndrome: If
You Think Feminism's Day Is Done, Just Ask the
Women Who've Made It." *This Magazine* 29, nos.
6/7 (March/April 1996): 26–29.

Mantilla, Karla. "An Hour of One's Own." *Off
Our Backs.* Retrieved from www.igc.org/oob/
features/worktime/feature03.htm (September 25,
2001).

———. "Women Who Work Too Much Fight
Back: Interview with Barbara Brant." *Off Our
Backs.* Retrieved from www.igc.org/oob/features/
worktime/feature01.htm (September 25, 2001).

McColl, Fiona. "Eight Easy Ways to Spot an
Emotional Manipulator." Heartless Bitches
International. Retrieved from www.
heartlessbitches.com/rants/eighteasyways.shtml
(2000).

McKay, Shona. "The Work-Family Conundrum."
Financial Post Magazine, December 1997, 78–81.
Illustration.

McLean, Candis "A More-Than-Full-Time Job:
Single Parents Face a Desperate Search for
Answers to the Problems of Family Break Up."
Alberta Report 25, no. 19 (April 27, 1998): 32–33.

———. "Look Who Doesn't Want a Divorce:
New Studies Indicate That Women Are First to
File, but Joint Custody Keeps Families Together"
[Brinig-Allen study]. *British Columbia Report* 10,
no. 5 (January 11, 1999): 32–34.

Messing, Karen. "Women's Occupational Health
and Androcentric Science." *Canadian Woman
Studies* 14, no. 3 (Summer 1994): 11–16.
Bibliography.

Mighty E. Joy, and Lori E. Leach. "Bumps along
the Road: Survivors of Domestic Violence Share
Their Workplace Experiences." *Canadian Woman
Studies* 18, no. 1 (Spring 1998): 92–96.

"Migraines." Posted to www.migraines.org;
retrieved October 18, 2001.

Milstone, Carol. "How to Save Your Marriage"
[emotionally focused couples therapy]. *Saturday
Night* 115, no. 10 (July 8, 2000): 32–39.
Illustrations.

Monhan Bartel, Margaret. "The Woods in
Winter: Hiking as Stress Therapy." *Country
Living* 17, no. 2 (February 1994): 65.

Mooy, Johanna M., et al. "Major Stressful Life
Events in Relation to Prevalence of Undetected

Type 2 Diabetes." *Diabetes Care* 23, no. 2 (February 2000): 197.

"More Vacation Spas Set Men and Women on Road to Wellness: Stress Is the Prime Reason for Attending a Wellness Spa." Canadian Press newswire, July 26, 1995.

Morrison, Judith H. The Book of Ayurveda. New York: Simon and Schuster: 1995.

Murphy, Lisa. "Is Work Hurting Your Health?" *Chatelaine* 73, no. 11 (November 2000): 66–75.

———. "The Love Test [taking your relationship in for a once-over]." *Chatelaine* 74, no. 2 (February 2001): 95–99.

Namie, Dr. Ruth, and Dr. Gary Namie. "Are You Exposed to Workplace Bullying/Are You the Bully." *Vicit Vim Virtus.* Retrieved from www.gojobrights.com/Articles/19990815vol2Bullytactics.html (August 1999).

National Advisory Committee on Immunization (NACI). "An Advisory Committee Statement (ACS) on Influenza Vaccination for the 2001–2002 Season." *Canada Communicable Disease Report,* 27 ACS-41 (August 2001).

National Association of Working Women. "Executive Summary: Investigative Report on Discriminatory Hiring Practices in Temporary Employment Agencies." *9 to 5.* Retrieved from www.9to5.org/newsf.html#temp (September 25, 2001).

———. "Facts on Working Women's Issues." *9 to 5.* Retrieved from www.9to5.org/facts.html (September 25, 2001).

Nicolaides, Carole. "Advantages of Being a Woman Entrepreneur." Retrieved online from www.allthatwomenwant.com/advantagewoman.htm (September 25, 2001).

Oliva, Robert M. "Meditation: A Great Way to Deal with Stress." *Self-Help for Her.* Retrieved online from www.selfhelpforher.com/innerjourney28.htm.

Ontario Task Force on the Primary Prevention of Cancer. *Recommendations for the Primary Prevention of Cancer: Report of the Ontario Task Force on the Primary Prevention of Cancer.* Toronto, March 1995.

"Out of the Shadows: Policy Principles to Recognize Women's Unpaid Work" [first part of full text]. *Economic Justice Report* 8, no. 3 (October 1997): 1–8.

Pierpont, Margaret, and Tegmeyer, Diane. *The Spa Life at Home.* Vancouver: Whitecap Books, 1997.

"Pilates." Retrieved from www.oprah.com (September 25, 2001).

Pirisi, Angela. "Alcohol's Siege on Women's Health." *Journal of Addiction and Mental Health* 3, no. 3 (May/June 2000): 13.

Pittaway, Tina. "100 Top Women Entrepreneurs." *Chatelaine* 72, no. 11 (November 1999): 72–78.

Pozner, Jennifer L. "One Giant Step for a Woman, One Small Step for Womankind." *Feminista!* 3, no. 9 (March 2000), www.feminista.com/v3n9/pozner.html.

———. "Why Reporters Talk to White Guys in Suits." *Feminista!* 3, no. 9 (March 2000), www.feminista.com/v3n9/pozner2.html.

"Profiles of Three Women in Poverty." Retrieved from www.oprah.com (September 25, 2001).

Reing, Michael. "Stress and Genital Herpes Recurrences in Women." *Journal of the American Medical Association* 283, no. 11 (March 15, 2000): 1394.

"Researcher Calls for Policy Measures to Cut Stigma of Women's Drinking." *Journal* (Addiction Research Foundation) 25, no. 3 (May/June 1996): 7.

Resinger, Monica. "A Decision to Stay Home." *All That Women Want.* Retrieved from www.allthatwomenwant.com/stayhome.htm (September 25, 2001).

Rich, Pat. "Women Doctors Juggle Too Much: Stress and Fatigue Levels Too High, Psychiatrist Says." *Medical Post* 35, no. 29 (September 7, 1999): 13. Illustrations.

Roberts, Francine M. *The Therapy Sourcebook.* Chicago: NTC/Contemporary Publishing, 1998.

Rosen, Larry, and Michelle M. Weil. *Technostress: Coping With Technology@Work @Home @Play.* New York: John Wiley & Sons, 1997.

Rosenthal, M. Sara. *The Canadian Type 2 Diabetes Sourcebook.* Toronto: Macmillan Canada, 2002.

———. *50 Ways to Manage Stress.* Chicago: Contemporary Books/McGraw-Hill, 2001.

———. *The Gastrointestinal Sourcebook.* Los Angeles: Lowell House, 1997.

———. "Imagine Community Ethics Taking Centre Stage." Paper presented at the 13th Annual Conference and Meeting, The Canadian Bioethics Society, Winnipeg, Manitoba, October 11-14, 2001

———. *Women and Depression.* Los Angeles: Lowell House, 2000.

———. *Women of the '60s Turning 50.* Toronto: Prentice Hall Canada, 2000.

———. *Women and Passion.* Toronto: Prentice Hall Canada: 2000.

Rowland, Rhonda. "Natural Cures for the Common Cold?" Retrieved from cnn.com (February 13, 2001).

Sangster, Joan. "Women and Work Assessing Canadian Women's Labour History at the Millenium." *Atlantis* 25, no. 1 (Fall 2000).

Schamer, Linda A., and Michael J Jackson. "Coping with Stress: Common Sense about Teacher Burnout." *Education Canada* 36, no. 2 (Summer 1996): 28–31.

Seldon, Zéna, and Dawn Farough. "Rough Answers: Abiding Concerns about Gender Discrimination and Access to Mortgage Funding." *Atlantis* 23, no. 2 (Spring 1999).

Seymour, Rhea, "Herpes Alert." *Chatelaine* 73, no. 2 (February 2000): 46.

"Shopping Addiction." Retrieved from www.oprah.com (September 25, 2001).

Side, Katherine. "Government Restraint and Limits to Economic Reciprocity in Women's Friendships." *Atlantis* 23, no. 2 (Spring 1999).

Smereka, Corinne M. "Outwitting, Controlling Stress for a Healthier Lifestyle." *Healthcare Financial Management* 44, no. 3 (March 1990): 70(5).

Smid, Madelon. "Beware of Illusory Freedom: The Simultaneous Rise in Women's Stress and Female Business May Be Related." *Report Newsmagazine* 26, no. 49 (March 13, 2000): 44–45.

Smith, Sandra, et. al. "Experiencing the Glass Ceiling." *Shatter the Glass Ceiling.* Retrieved from www. theglassceiling.com/glass/ww1_34.htm (June 25, 1999).

"Sources of Stress in Unemployed Female Managers: An Exploratory Study" [Part 2 of 4]. *International Review of Women and Leadership* 2, no. 2 (December 1996).

"Sources of Stress in Unemployed Female Managers: An Exploratory Study" [Part 3 of 4]. *International Review of Women and Leadership* 2, no. 2 (December 1996).

Spiker, Ted. "Choose to Snooze." *Men's Health* 15, no. 4 (May 2000): 56.

Spivak, Diane. "Hey, Aren't You Whatsisface?" *Chatelaine* 73, no. 11 (November 2000): 91–97.

Steinem, Gloria, *Revolution from Within: A Book of Self-Esteem.* New York: Little, Brown and Company: 1992, 1993.

Stier, J.J. "A Boon for Whom." *Feminista!* 4, no. 2. Retrieved from www.feminista.com/v4n2/stier.html (September 25, 2001).

"Stress May Intensify Cold Symptoms." Posted online to www.mediconsult.com (March 26, 1999).

"Stress Test." Retrieved from www.oprah.com (September 25, 2001).

"Stress-Busters: What Works." *Newsweek International,* June 28, 1999, 52.

Teish, Luisah. "Big Mommas and Golden Apples." *Ms. Magazine,* October/November 1999.

Time Health Media Inc. "Alcohol abuse." *Health.* Retrieved from www.health.com/wykns/ Alcohol_AbuseWYNK2000-MAL/whatisit.html (September 25, 2001).

Time Health Media Inc. "What You Can Do to Quit Smoking." *Health.* Retrieved from www. health.com/wykns/SmokingWYNK2000-MAL/whatyoucando.html (September 25, 2001).

"Tobacco: A Menace to Women's Health." *Women in Action* 3, no. 3 (1998): 68.

"Up in Smoke: Why Teen Girls Don't Quit." *Chatelaine* 69, no. 7 (July 1996): 29–33.

U.S. Department of Labor Office of Public Affairs. "Report from the Glass Ceiling Commission." *Shatter the Glass Ceiling,* www.theglassceiling.com/glass/ww2_repo.htm.

U.S. Department of Labor Office of the Secretary Women's Bureau. "A Working Woman's Guide to Her Rights." *Shatter the Glass Ceiling,* www.theglassceiling.com/wib2/ww2_work.htm.

———. "Family and Medical Leave—Know Your Rights." *Shatter the Glass Ceiling,* www.theglassceiling.com/wib2/ww_17fam.htm.

Vaughn, Debra. "Top 10 Reasons People Over Spend." *All That Women Want,* www. allthatwomenwant.com/overspend.htm (2001).

Vaz-Oxlade, Gail E. "A Woman's Darkest Fear: Widowhood." *Chatelaine* 73, no. 10 (October 2000): 50.

Watts, Suzanne. "A Girl's Guide to Avoiding the Emotional Blackmailer." Heartless Bitches International. Retrieved from www.heartlessbitches.com/rants/black2.shtml.

"What Is It about Women and Guilt?" *Chatelaine* 66, no. 4 (April 1993): 55–57.

"What to Do When You're out of Work." Retrieved from www.oprah.com (September 25, 2001).

Whitty, Claire, Bach Flower Remedy practitioner. Posted to www.gofree.indigo.ie/ ~bachflwr/index.htm; retrieved October 22, 2001.

"Who's the Typical Canadian Mom?" [survey]. *Chatelaine* 67, no. 5 (May 1994): 41–45.

"Why Women Experience More Depression Than Men Do." *Today's Woman.* Retrieved from www.todayswoman.com/depression.html (September 25, 2001).

Wolf, Naomi. *Misconceptions.* New York: Doubleday, 2001.

"A Woman's Lifetime Guide to Financial Security." *Chatelaine* 67, no. 3 (March 1994): 47–49.

"Women Gamblers Increasing." Canadian Press newswire, April 17, 1996.

"Women Hit Harder by Welfare Reforms" [four women challenging spouse-in-the-house regulation]. Canadian Press newswire, June 11, 1996.

"Women in Debt." Women's Financial Network (WFN) at Siebert. Retrieved from www.wfn.com/ pages/page.asp?pageID=169&SID=8&ArticleID= 623& ishome=1 (September 25, 2001).

"Women's Alcohol Consumption Is Up." *Marketing to Women* 13, no. 10 (October 2000): 3.

"The Work-Family Crunch: How Are We Coping?" [results of a readers' survey]. *Chatelaine* 69, no. 4 (April 1996): 55–59.

"Writing about Stress Improves Your Health." *Research Digest.* Posted to www.mediconsult.com (June 16, 1999).

Zellerbach, Merla. *The Allergy Sourcebook.* Los Angeles: Lowell House, 1995.

Zeytinoglu, Isik U., and Jacinta K. Muteshi. "A Critical Review of Flexible Labour: Gender, Race and Class Dimensions of Economic Restructuring" [second part of full text]. *Resources for Feminist Research* 27, nos. 3/4 (Fall 1999/Winter 2000): 97–120.

Index

A

Aboriginal women, and domestic violence, 127

ace-inhibitors, 44

acupuncture, 194; for stopping smoking, 91

acute stress, 134

addictions: to alcohol, 93–96; to drugs, 101–104; endorphins and, 87; gambling, 147; shopping, 133–34; smoking, 83–92; to spending, 146–47

adrenaline, and chronic fatigue syndrome, 40

aging, 158–62

agism, 132

alcohol: addiction, 93–96; and high blood pressure, 42; intake and headaches, 19; and PMS, 96; and weight gain, 96

Alcoholics Anonymous, 93, 94, 100

Alexander technique, 196

Alexander, Frederick Matthias, 196

allergies, viii, 13–16; and autoimmune system, 13; and fatigue, 13–14; herbal treatments for, 15–16; treating with over-the-counter medications, 16; triggers, 20

alpha-blocking agents, 44

ambivalence, 68

American Holistic Nurses Association, 191

American Massage Therapy Association, 192

American Psychiatric Association, 64, 65

Anderson, Carol, 124

anger: and bullying, 139; in relationships, 124–27; unexpressed, 139

anhedonia, 63

anorexia nervosa, 101, 151–52, 154

antibiotics, and bacterial sinusitis, 7–8

anticholinergics, as cold treatment, 10

antidepressants, vii, 66; and chronic fatigue syndrome, 41

antihistamines, 16

anti-inflammatory drugs, for colds, 9

anxiety, 50–58; about health, 57–58; about terrorism, 54–55; compared to worry, 54–55; generalized anxiety disorder, 53–55; managing, 57; in relationships, 51–53; in workplace, 53

assertiveness, 68

asthma attacks, 8

asthma, viii, 13–16; and fatigue, 13–14; in childhood, 36

astragalus, 201

autoimmune system, and allergies, 13

B

babysitters, 113

Bach flower remedies, 201–203

Bach, Edward, 201

back pain, viii

back rub instructions, 198

Baird, Zoe, 114

Balancing Act (book), 135

banks, sexist lending policies, 134, 144

bathroom, frequency of use, 25–26

bathroom-related stress, 25

beauty, unrealistic standards, 68

behavioural counselling, 90

beta carotene, 208

beta-blockers, 44

binge eating, 98–101, 154

bioflavonoids, 210

birthday survival tips, 188

bladder control, exercises for, 32

bladder problems, 30–32; and fibromyalgia, 39; improving control, 31–32

blood pressure, lowering, 206–207

blood sugar: and diabetes, 33; low, and panic attacks, 56

blood, in stool, 28

body image, 148–55

boron, 210

brain chemistry, 66; and depression, 64

breathing: exercises, 217–18; and life energy, 215–19

bronchitis, chronic, 8

Brook, Paula, 115

bulimia nervosa, 151–52, 154

bulimia, 100–101

bullying, in the workplace, 138–40, 141

burnout, 3, 36; symptoms of, ix

Burton, Linda, 114

businesses, starting, 144–45

C

caffeine, effects of overuse, 97–98

calcium, 210

calcium-channel blockers, 44

Campbell, Kim, 142

Canadian Mortgage and Housing Corporation, 145

cancer: and alcohol intake, 95; and autoimmune disease, 6; and car exhaust, 180; smoking and, 84

car exhaust, and cancer, 180

car, living without, 186

cardamom, 207

cardiovascular disease, 41–48; high blood pressure, 41–44; preventing, 47

careers; enjoying, 176–81; and families, 135, 136–38; stresses caused by, 110–14; working conditions, 137–38

caregiving: as cause of burnout, ix–x; for elderly parents, 118–20, 159; source of stress, 107

carotenes, 210

Carson, Rachel, 51

cayenne, 208

cellphone, restricting use of, 183

centrally acting agents, 44

Chatters, David, 137

chemical sensitivities, 14–15

chicken soup, Sara's, 10–11

child care, 106; choices, 112–13; policies in Europe, 137

children: birthday survival tips, 188; caring for, and fatigue, 35–36; delaying having, 188–89; and time management, 187–88

chiropracty, 193

Chopra, Deepak, 121, 180

chromium, 211

chronic fatigue, 13

chronic fatigue syndrome: and adrenaline, 40; and antidepressants, 41; causes, 39–40; and depression, 36; diet and, 40; and sleep disorders, 40; symptoms, 36–38; treatments, 40–41; trigger foods, 40

chronic stress, 134

cigarette smoke, and headache, 20

cigarettes, 83–92; "light," 88; as reward, 89

cigars, dangers of smoking, 92

cinnamon, 207

class, social, and weight, 150

Clinton, Bill, 113–14

clove, 207

cocaine, use of, 102–104

cognitive behavioural therapy, 57

colds: and asthma attacks, 8; avoiding, 8–9; and chronic bronchitis, 8; and cough suppressants, 10; ear infections, 8; preventing with echinacea, 8–9; related to stress, 7–11; sinus infections, 7–8; treating with anticholinergics, 10; treating with anti-inflammatory drugs, 9; treating with chicken soup, 10–11; treating with decongestants, 9–10; treating with over-the-counter medicines, 9–11; treating with zinc, 8

community family services, 71

commuting, reducing, 179–80

concentration, and depression, 62

constipation, irritable bowel syndrome, 26–27, 28

control, and food, 152

copper, 211

coriander, 207

cortisol, and fatigue, 35

cough suppressants, and cold treatments, 10

Coumadin, 48

counselling: for relationships, 131; grief, 171

counsellors, 71, 74–75, 90

Couple Enrichment Approach, 131

Couple Enrichment Inc., 120

crack cocaine, 103

creativity, nurturing, 220–21

credit cards, reducing, 185–86

crisis counsellors, 71

Crittenden, Danielle, 111

cross-addiction, 95

crying, importance of, 226

cumin, 207

Cyrenne, Huguette, 137

D

The Dance of Anger (book), 126

dandelion root, 43, 206

day care: policies in Europe, 137; types, 113

death, grieving process, 166–71

debt: reducing, 186–87; and women, 145–47

decongestants, for colds, 9–10

Deloitte & Touche, 137

depression, viii, ix; and anger, 125; bipolar, 58; brain chemistry and, 64; causes, 63–65; and chronic fatigue syndrome, 36; compared to sadness, 59–61; effect on concentration, 62; effect on sleep patterns, 62; employee assistance program for therapy, 70–71; family support during, 69; and grief, 169–70; herbal treatments for, 65–66; link with genetics, 64–65; loss of pleasure, 63; managing, 65–69; postpartum, 108–10; related to stress, 58–69; situational, 58; support groups, 66–69; symptoms, 61–63; therapy for, 70–82; treating with antidepressants, 66; treating with herbs, 200–201; unipolar, 58

diabetes: and blood sugar, 33; symptoms, 33–34; Type 1, and weight control, 151; Type 2, 33

diarrhea, and irritable bowel syndrome, 26–27, 28

diet supplements, 213–14

diet: and high blood pressure, 42; and stress, 96–104

digestion, improving, 207–208

digestive disorders, viii; and irritable bowel syndrome, 27

Dittmer, Janet, 114

diuretics, 43–44

divorce, 163–66

dogs, benefits of owning, 224

domestic violence, 127–28

Dorfman, Louise, 120, 121, 123, 131

downshifting, 176–89

drugs: abusing, 101–104; addiction to, 101–104; illegal, 102, 104; for lowering high blood pressure, 43–44; prescription, 102; for stopping smoking, 91–92

E

ear infections, 8

eating disorders, 98–101, 148, 151–52, 154; manifestation of anger, 125

echinacea: as cold treatment, 8–9; for strengthening immune system, 16–17

ecofeminism, 51

Ecstacy, use of, 103

education, for women, 143

emotional stress, viii

employee assistance program, 70–71

endorphins, and smoking, 87

energy healing, 191

energy, eliminating drains on, 184–85

Epstein-Barr virus, 36 See also Chronic fatigue syndrome

essential fatty acids, 210

essential oils, 203

Essiac, for strengthening immune system, 17

e-stress, reducing, 181–84

estrogen, 161; loss, and heart attacks, 45

exercise tolerance, 37

exercise: excessive, 151; and high blood pressure, 42

exercises: bladder control, 32; deep breathing, 217–18; meditative stretching, 218–19

exhaustion See Fatigue

F

families, and careers, 135, 136–38

family counsellors, 74–75

family life, 106

fatigue, viii, ix See also Chronic fatigue syndrome; and allergies, 13–14; and asthma, 13–14; and caring for children, 35–36; and headaches, 18; role of cortisol, 35; and stress, 34–41

Feldenkrais method, 196–97

Feldenkrais, Moshe, 196

feminism, 111, 136, 143

feminist therapy, 79–81

feng shui, 222

fennel, 207

fibromyalgia, 36 See also Chronic fatigue syndrome; and irritable bowel syndrome, 39

finances, restructuring, 186–87

financial security, 134

Fiorina, Carleton, 142

Fitzgerald, William, 195

flirting, 140–41

flower remedies, 201–203

flu, 11–13; and immune system, 11; homeopathic treatments, 12; symptoms, 12; vaccine, 11, 12

Flying Solo (book), 124

folic acid, 210

food banks, 146

food: and control, 152; importance of enjoying, 225–26; for reducing stress, 208–14; relationship to stress, 96–104

forgiveness, 226

Friedan, Betty, 107, 108

friends, importance of, 171–73

functional bowel disorder *See* Irritable bowel syndrome

G

gadgets, limiting use of, 183

gambling, 147

garlic, 43, 207

gender economics, 134

generalized anxiety disorder, 53–55

genetics, link to depression, 64–65

ginger, 207

ginkgo, 201

ginseng, 43, 201, 207; for strengthening immune system, 17

glass ceiling syndrome, 141–43

green tea, for strengthening immune system, 17

grief counsellors, 171

grief, 166–71; and depression, 169–70

gynecological problems, 158

H

Habitrol, 90

Hanson, Jennifer, 137

hawthorn, 43, 206

Hay, Louise, 121

headaches, viii, 18–24; and alcohol intake, 19; and cigarette smoke, 20; cluster, 19; and fatigue, 18; herbal treatment for, 20; medication causing, 21; at menopause, 18; and menstrual cycle, 22; migraine, 22–24; and pregnancy, 18; rebound, 20–21; recording in diary, 24; secondary, 21–22; sinus, 20; and sleep patterns, 19; and smoking, 19; tension, 18–19; triggers of migraine, 23–24; and weather changes, 19

healers, hands-on, 197–98

Health Canada, 97

health, anxiety about, 57–58

heart, herbs for strengthening, 205–207

heart attack: lowering risk, 206–207; risk of, 5; recovering from, 46; symptoms in women, 45–46; in women, 44–45

Henrik, Per, 192

herbal remedies: for incontinence, 31–32; to lower high blood pressure, 43

herbal treatments: for allergies, 15–16; for colds, 8–9; for depression, 65–66; for headache, 20; for the heart, 205–207; for panic attacks, 205–206; for reducing stress, 199–204; for stopping smoking, 90; strengthening immune system, 16–18

Hewlett-Packard, 142

high blood pressure, viii, 41–44; herbal remedies, 43; lowering with drugs, 43–44; lowering without drugs, 42–43

Hite, Shere, 135, 140

homeopathic treatments: for flu, 12–13; for stopping smoking, 90

hormone replacement therapy, 161; treating incontinence, 32

hospitals, therapy for depression in, 71

housework, conflict over, 117–18

hypertension, 42

hypnosis, for stopping smoking, 91

hypoglycemia, 97

I

immune suppression, viii; related to stress, 6–18

immune system: and flu, 11; strengthening, 16–18; and stress, viii, 2

incontinence, 25, 31–32; conventional remedies for, 32; herbal remedies for, 31–32

influenza *See* Flu

insulin resistance, and stress, 32–34

Internet, limiting use of, 183

interstitial cystitis, 30

iron, 211

irritable bowel syndrome, 25–30; and fibromyalgia, 39; and stress, 29; and women, 30; symptoms, 27–28

iscador, for strengthening immune system, 17

ischemia, 46

ischemic stroke, 47

K

karoshi, 4

kava root, 200

Keen, Sam, 129

Kegel exercises, 32

physical conditions related to stress, 2–3

physical stress, viii

physical symptoms of panic attacks, vii

pink ghetto, ix

pleasure, loss of, and depression, 63

PMS, 48–49; and alcohol intake, 96

postpartum depression, 108–10

posture, improving, 196–97

potassium, 43, 207, 212

poverty, and women, 145–47

powerlessness, 68

pregnancies

pregnancy, 157–58; and autoimmune disease, 6; and headaches, 18; postpartum depression, 108–10; and working conditions, 15

premenstrual discomforts, 156–57

premenstrual syndrome *See* PMS

pressure point therapy, 194–96

pressure points, self-massage, 195–96

privacy, lack of, 182

Prozac, 200

psychiatric nurses, 74

psychiatrists, 73

psychoanalysis, 81–82

psychological associates, 73

psychologists, 73

psychotherapy *See* Therapy

pyridoxne, 210

Q

qi gong, 216–17

R

reflexology, 195

relationships, 120–31; anger in, 124–27; with body, 149; counselling, 131; defined, 123; with mother, 153; negative, 124–31

Reno, Janet, 114

reproductive concerns, 15

Rescue Remedy, 201–202

retirement funds, using to reduce debt, 186

rheumatism, 36 *See also* Chronic fatigue syndrome

riboflavin, 209

Rolf, Ida, 197

Rolfing, 197

Royal Bank of Canada, 138

Rubinstein, David, 120, 121, 123, 131

S

sabbatical leave, 181

sadness, compared to depression, 59–61

St. John's wort, 65–66, 200

St. Lewis, Joanne, 143

Sam-e, 200

Schultz, Sigrid, 51

seaweed, 43, 207

selenium, 212

self-care, 220–26

self-employment, 144–45

self-esteem, 150

self-financing, 144–45

self-harm, 125

self-worth, 150

Selye, Hans, 2

Sex and Business (book), 135

Sex and the City (TV show), 134

sexism, 67

sexual harassment, 140–41

Sheehy, Gail, 160

shiatsu, 192, 195

Shoman, Mary J., 6

shopping, addiction to, 133–34

Silent Spring (book), 51

silicon, 212

single mothers, 137, 146

sinus infections, 7–8

sleep deprivation, 34–36

sleep disorders, and chronic fatigue syndrome, 40

sleep patterns, and depression, 62

sleep, appropriate levels, 35

Smith's Pharmacy, 12, 90

smoking, 83–92; and cancer, 84; endorphins and, 87; and headaches, 19; quitting, 87, 89–92; as reward, 89; starting, 88

social workers, 74

spending, controlling, 186–87

spending addictions, 146–47

spending habits, 133–34

spices, counteracting tumours, 17–18

spouse, death of, 166–71

Steinem, Gloria, 128, 129, 149

Stewart, Martha, 220

Stewart, Susan, 124

stress hormones, 2

stress: acute, 4; chronic, 4, 5; definition, 2; reducing, 181–87; symptoms of, 2–3, 4; types of, 4–5

stretching, 218–19

stroke: lowering risk, 206–207; risk of, 5; symptoms, 48; and women, 47–48

sulfur, 212

Supermom, 106, 115–17

Superwoman myth, 111

support groups, for depression, 66–69

surfing, limiting time, 183

Swedish massage, 192

T

technology, stress of, 181–84

telecommuting, 179

terrorism, anxiety about, 54–55

therapists: age of, 77; choosing, 75–77; credentials, 72–75; crisis counsellors, 71; fees, 75; friends' recommendations, 71–72; how to find, 70–72; lifestyle of, 77; private, 72

therapy: biologically informed, 78; cognitive-behavioural, 78–79; community family services, 71; for depression, 70–82; employee assistance program, 70–71; feminist, 79–81; interpersonal, 81; pressure point, 194–96; psychoanalysis, 81–82; psychodynamic, 82; styles, 77–82; women's health clinics, 71

thiamine, 209

thyroid disease, 6

tobacco industry, 85–86

tobacco, contents of smoke, 88–89

toilet schedules, 32

Trager method, 197

Trager, Milton, 197

turmeric, 207

Turner, John, 142

Type A personality, and stress, 4

V

vacation time, 181

valerian root, 201

Valium, 102

vasodilators, 44

vertigo, vii, viii

violence, domestic, 127–28

vitamin A, 208

vitamin B$_1$, 209

vitamin B$_{12}$, 209

vitamin B$_2$, 209

vitamin B$_6$, 208

vitamin C, 209

vitamin D, 209

vitamin E, 209

vitamin K, 209

W

weather, and headaches, 19, 23–24

weight control, 148–55

weight gain, and alcohol intake, 96

West, Mae, 150

What's a Smart Girl Like You Doing at Home? (book), 114

wheatgrass, for strengthening immune system, 17

Winfrey, Oprah, 220

Wolf, Naomi, 107, 108, 109, 110, 111, 114, 117

women of colour, 143

women's health clinics, 71

Women's Legal Education Action Fund (LEAF), 143

work life: enjoying, 176–81; and stress, 110–14

working conditions, 137–38; affecting pregnancies, 15

Working Mother Magazine, 143

Working Woman Magazine, 143

workplace, stress in, 132

workplace bullying, 138–40, 141

workplace chemicals, dangers of, 13

workplace hazards, 15

workweek, reducing, 180

Y

Yaccato, Joanne Thomas, 135

yoga, 215–16

Z

Zicam (zinc nasal spray), 9

zinc nasal spray, 9

zinc, 212; as cold treatment, 8

Zyban, 91, 92